TOSS OF THE COIN
Choosing My Gay Destiny

TOSS OF THE COIN
Choosing My Gay Destiny

ROB TACKES
An Audacious Memoir

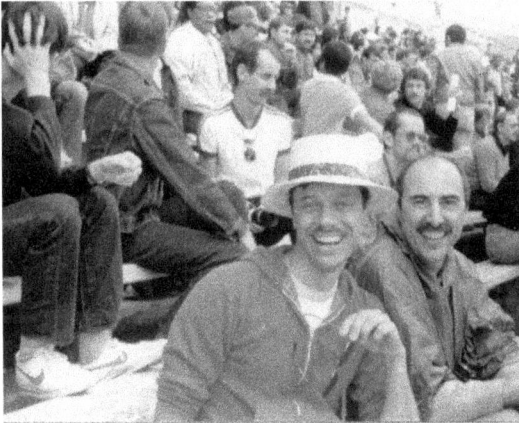

Rob and Denis at first Gay Games, Kezar Stadium, S.F., 1982.

Rob Tackes was a shy, gay youth exploring Chicago in the 1940s and 50s. He and his partner Denis moved to San Francisco at the start of the gay revolution.

Rob's spirited experiences included escapades in real estate, mariquana, and sex. HIV hit him hard in 1981, but through persistence he became a miracle long-term survivor.

Rob and Denis currently live in Palm Springs, California.

Desert Muse Books
Palm Springs
desertmusebooks.com

Toss of the Coin: Choosing My Gay Destiny
Copyright © 2017 Rob Tackes

Paperback: ISBN 978-0-9985622-1-6
E-Book:　　ISBN 978-0-9985622-0-9
Library of Congress Control Number: 2017900528

Publisher's Cataloging-in-Publication Data
provided by Five Rainbows Cataloging Services:
Names: Tackes, Rob.
Title: Toss of the coin : choosing my gay destiny, an audacious memoir / Rob Tackes.
Description: Palm Springs : Desert Muse Books, 2017. | Includes bibliographical references.
Identifiers: LCCN 2017900528 | ISBN 978-0-9985622-1-6 (pbk.) | ISBN 978-0-9985622-0-9 (ebook)
Subjects: LCSH: Gay men--Biography. | HIV-positive gay men--Biography. | San Francisco (Calif.)--Biography. | Chicago (Ill.)--Biography. | Love. | BISAC: BIOGRAPHY & AUTOBIOGRAPHY / LGBT. | BIOGRAPHY & AUTOBIOGRAPHY / Personal Memoirs.
Classification: LCC HQ75.8.T33 A3 2017 (print) | LCC HQ75.8.T33 (ebook) | DDC 306.766/2--dc23.

Published in the United States by
Desert Muse Books
Palm Springs, CA
Website desertmusebooks.com
Email memoir@desertmusebooks.com

Cover design by Linda Kosarin
Editing by Don Weise

Printed in the United States of America

Distributed through Querelle/Independent

For Denis
Your unconditional love has set me
Free

Here is what *He* had to say on my 74th birthday.

Today is so rare,
Start floating on air!
Come out with a roar,
It's seventy-four

Love, D.

Tra La, Tra La, Tra La.
Everyone else is talking about men.
They want one.
Tra La
I've got one!

Rob.

CONTENTS

The author has set up a website for additional material, including extended commentary and a huge folio of photos, plus posters from the 1970s:

Website desertmusebooks.com
Email memoir@desertmusebooks.com

Why did I write this book?
Why should you read it?

This memoir is dedicated to all the men dealing with their sexual identity, to give them some valuable history and support them in their unique coming out process.

My memories and anecdotes of life in times gone by will clue them and help them navigate through their own special needs.

All of us can surmount the gross generalizations often present in society about gay people. We have the ability to create an honest, civilized dialogue with those around us.

Finally, my unique experiences can be a helpful reference point for parents, grandparents, family and friends. My story will alert them to the special situations and the mindsets of gay men who are successful, happy and fulfilled.

The author is in Palm Springs, looking back at his life and realizing that most people today seem to lack curiosity, don't question authority, and blindly accept mainstream distortions rampant in our society.

Why am I different?
How did I develop a vibrant life based on a triangle of priorities?
Here is my story ...

PROLOGUE
The best of times. The worst of times

"It was the turn of the 21st century. San Francisco, the big City, continued to exert its charms, offering loads of opportunities for me to meet interesting people at bars, beaches, cafés and at the most creative sex clubs.

I'm having another night out at my favorite venue for sex. A hit or two of cannabis sets my mood. After checking in, I begin the parade through mazes, cubicles and ramps to access willing men. I am seeking a sensual Nirvana, as are all the men here.

A little blue pill has helped me enhance my libido but unfortunately it also brings a smoky blue haze to my eyes in the half darkness. Feeling odd and woozy I sit down in the television room on a high wooden step.

Boing! I Pass out for a moment and fall forward and down onto the cement floor. There is a gash on my head above my eye but the fall brings me back to consciousness. Blood, then first aid and a shocked recovery, a drive home, then to sleep. It is a fair warning.

Never again, well hardly ever again, would I be seeking this kind of excess."

My saga had begun much earlier …

PART ONE

MY EARLY LIFE
A History of the Era

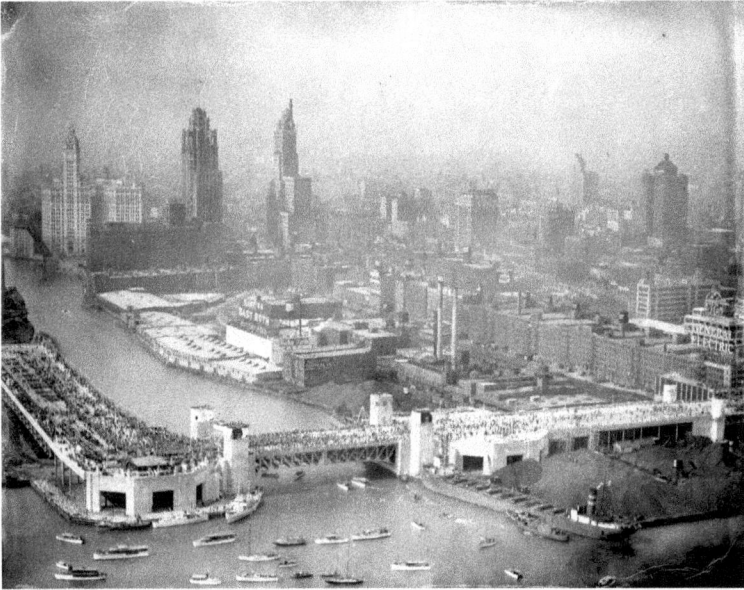

Chicago, 1937. My roots. A powerhouse city.
A cultural and economic giant.

Adventures in Urban Mid-Century America

1. MY EARLY LIFE IN CHICAGO

There was an awakening in me at age five. My cousin Quentin was in the navy and he stayed with us for a few nights and slept with me in my double bed. As he came home late one night I caught him undressing and was fascinated as I peeked at his skivvies. The second night he was having nightmares and started smothering me with his pillow. I was so afraid to say something to resist. Finally, I cried out "Stop." Oh, what a scare.

My beginning was on February 6, 1937. Mom was relieved that cold February morning when Bobby popped out a beautiful, healthy baby. What incredible blue eyes, bluer and lighter than dads. Mom was twenty-five and dad thirty-two. It meant that their carefree life was ending and they had to adjust to me as their new responsibility. Mom was a quiet one compared to her sisters and brother, also the most conservative. Very much like her mother, Mary. Dad was a farmer's son, a fish out of water in the big city, and supposedly a spoiled youth, the youngest of nine.

Dad early on told me that I shared that February sixth birthday with Babe Ruth. Strangely I have never had an athletic bone in my body. Dad nevertheless was proud of the connection.

1937 was a big year for other reasons than my birth. The Hindenburg exploded, Europe was falling apart, Amelia Earhart disappeared, and King Edward VIII married the divorced Wallis Simpson. *Snow White and the Seven Dwarfs* came out on the movie screen. A sign of things to come in my life?

After my delivery at the hospital I took up residence in a basement apartment on Belmont Avenue on Chicago's near Northwest Side.

Mom, Dad and I lived in the three-flat building that my mother's parents, the Ascherls, had purchased new in 1915. Grandpa and Grandma lived on top. Dad had just been called back to his switchboard testing job at Western Electric after having been laid off when the Great Depression took hold in the early 1930s. He now had a steady income again. As a single man, to tide himself through the Depression, he had slung hash at the Hungarian pavilion at Chicago's Century of Progress in 1932. He also worked at other temporary jobs in the 1930s including hard work on the railroad. My mom was a homemaker who had been a stenographer during those trying times.

In 1939 we moved out of the damp basement apartment and up to the middle flat out of concern for my health. That December my brother Tommy was born. I was moved from a cozy spot in my parent's room to the second bedroom to make way. It was a mild shock to be alone at night. I had many a nightmare alone in my own bedroom until I got used to being by myself. I did enjoy those early dreams that included me flying above danger. I learned to control myself in my dreams and could come out of scary events by forcing myself to wake up. Unfortunately, those dreams of imaginative flights of fancy and my control over them disappeared when I got older. Perhaps because the real world became more of a concern to me and my fanciful early childhood juices were put on hold.

Another of my earliest remembrances was in Delavan, Wisconsin, at my grandparent's summer cottage. There I was, on our folding cot, under the old maple tree, naked with my butt in the air. I have a photo to prove it. I also remember a darkened room in my baby bed with the side guards up where I languished with the measles. I actually loved being in and around enclosures. A tub here and a playpen there, were my secure zones.

February 1942 was my first day of kindergarten. My mother thought that I was an intelligent child (of course), so she decided to enter me in school mid-year February when I turned five. It was traumatic for me. My classmates had already spent half the school year together and I was the new timid child tossed into the fray. I felt out of sync with the rest of the students and it took me awhile to calm down and to accept the initial fright of being with strangers. Only much later in life, when I discovered I had to be more aggressive to achieve my goals, did I realize that I had to make overt attempts to welcome "strangers."

When my youngest brother, Jerry, was born in 1944, I was quite amused by his red hair. For many months, I had accompanied my mother to her doctor's office while she was pregnant. Waiting with her seemed endless in that large waiting room filled with other expectant mothers. The reason for the wait was that most doctors were off to the war. From those interminable waits I acquired impatience, and since then I have always tried to get things done in a prompt and timely fashion.

During the war years, I was oblivious to the horrendous things happening in the world. I do remember the blackouts. We had to pull all our shades down to thwart the enemy from seeing our buildings and bombing us. We occasionally went upstairs during those blackouts to visit with my grandparents, where we sat around in the darken dining room lit by candles. Downstairs when we had blackout drills, my parents would sit in the dark on our living room sofa, and I snuggled up between them. I was hypnotized and enthralled with the eerie dance of the lights on our walls, that appeared each time a streetcar passed by outside.

The first visitors I remember where my father's nephews, who were in the military. They were passing through Chicago on their way to their military destinations. We rarely had out of town visitors so these visits lodged in my mind and became part of my first social situations. Interacting with these new faces was as uncomfortable for me as it was for my father, who I sensed was uneasy with the visitors, even though they were close relatives.

My first trauma came one day in the second grade at St. Francis elementary school when Sister Richardine caught me day dreaming, and she twisted my ear so hard that it burned. I turned a very hot red. As a result of this embarrassment I decided to never again be singled out. From that point onward I would toe the line and not make waves. Straight "A"s from now on was my goal, and excelling at school was my way to avoid being criticized.

It was the radio serials of the 1940s that sent me into my next flights of fancy. I was mesmerized listening to the dialogue and visualizing the characters in their scenes as flesh and blood. There I was, stretched on out my stomach, on the floor and savoring these sounds and images as my own.

2. CHILDHOOD IN THE COUNTRY

Delavan, Wisconsin during the war years was a kid's country delight. Delavan was a two-hour drive from Chicago out Route 14, the Northwest Highway. Dad drove our 1939 Plymouth at a maximum of 50 miles per hour to help save gas because we had to be careful not to exceed our allotments of gasoline mandated by the government. When we reached "the gravel road" we knew we were five minutes away from our destination. Grandma and Grandpa were there to greet us. We had arrived.

Those early trips often gave me a bit of car sickness, but the fun of the country made the trip worthwhile. On our broad lawns, I reveled inside my play pen, and later played with pots and barrels. I definitely had an affinity for these safely enclosed spaces. A battered, orange enamel basin intrigued me. I loved caressing that pot on the front porch, and at age one and one-half, my parents caught me on their brownie camera and cemented my cuteness. They said "smile" and I gave them an especially large one. This photo is one of my favorites and is on my mantle at home today.

In the summer of 1941 my grandparents hosted one very big country community gathering. Neighbors from the Lake Delavan Highlands subdivision and relatives, mainly from my grandfather's side of the family, gathered on our lawn to mingle, gossip, drink beer, pop and eat sausages. I was a shy 4-year-old, amazed by the crowd. It was overwhelming to little old me. Everyone seemed to be in a happy mood. *Gemütlichkeit*, for this overwhelmingly Germanic group. A group photograph was taken and recorded the essence of this party of almost 150 people. The war was around the corner, Hitler's move on Europe was already underway, and for one last time these people were going to have a hell of a good time. The photo shows one man raising his arm overseeing the crowd, who either was making fun of the oaf Hitler, or recording his admiration for him. I will never know.

A couple of years later, when I was six, our family organized a mushroom hunt. We faithfully walked up on the rutted gravel of Spruce Street, past the Capitol Ballroom at the corner, and on to the farm land attached to an imposing horse farm. The farm was owned by a Chicago mafia figure and Grandpa obtained his permission to gather mushrooms. On the search, I was assigned to my grandfather and was alone with him in the woods. We got lost and were separated from the rest of the group, and when the two of us came to a barbed wire fence blocking our path, Grandpa Ascherl swore "Damn it." I had never experienced strong language or anger up to that point. We had to jump over a barbed wire fence in order to locate and re-join the rest of the mushroom party. I don't remember if we found any mushrooms but I sure remember Grandpa's adult anger!

My grandfather, as a young man, lived in a Polish town in Austrian-controlled Galicia. Grandma told me that he spoke better Polish than German when she first met him. Grandpa, as I was told, had a "temper." I think that was code for something more complicated. Did he have a more sophisticated understanding of the contradictions and gyrations of world politics? Undoubtedly. Another mysterious bit of information that leaked out later was that he didn't like President Roosevelt. To me as a kid this was almost un-American. I have often wondered why he did not like Roosevelt. Was it Roosevelt's decision to get into the war with Germany? What else could it have been? Was it possible that my grandpa's sympathies were with "the Bund," a group in the United States that was heavily in favor of Hitler's success in reasserting Germany's power? Our usual tight lipped family never mentioned any more details about this.

In 1945 World War II ended. We heard the news first on the car radio. VE Day. I asked "What is that?" "Victory in Europe," my parents said. Soon there was a VJ Day, which stood for Victory over Japan in the Pacific. Strangely we also heard this news on our car radio coming home from Delevan.

3. "CATHOLICISM"

My best memories, about my early experiences in and around the Catholic Church, were the beauty of the ceremonies and the pageantry that took place inside our parish church, St. Francis Xavier. The side alters were dedicated to St. Joseph and to the Blessed Virgin Mary. I was overwhelmed by the majesty of the decorations covering those gothic wood altars, when they were decorated for Easter and Christmas. The flowers, the purple-colored bunting, the smell of incense, and the vaulted ceilings and stained glass windows overwhelmed me and filled me with awe.

But there were things about the Church I didn't like: Hard kneelers while saying the dreaded rosary, a long string of beads that require reciting prayers including, *Hail Mary's, Our Fathers and the Apostles Creed,* all while fingering each bead. Then there were the frightful, foreboding confessional rooms where we had to admit our flaws.

As neared seven, the age of reason, my first holy communion was imminent. Because I was always the shortest boy in my class, I was chosen lead the communion march down the center aisle of church. Conveniently I got sick the week before the event, but I was getting better and my parents allowed me to decide whether I wanted to go through with the ceremony with the rest of the class. I did not want the responsibility of being on view to lead the whole class down the aisle, so, pondering the situation I took the easy way out. "No," I told them. Several weeks later, when my class was in church, I stepped up to the plate and took my First Holy Communion separately, quietly. That was trauma enough.

Our church was a brick modified-Gothic edifice that had a thirty-two-bell carillon that was erected in the belfry in 1948. It was the pride of all the parishioners. The sounds could be heard for quite a distance, and depending on the wind we caught a whiff of the bells at our house.

Our rules were that we go to church every Sunday, and that we follow the church rule of meatless Fridays. I dutifully went to confession which was a particularly scary event for me. I did not think that I had committed any sins, so I made them up. "Father it has been two weeks since my last confession. I disobeyed my parents two times…" The penance was to say some prayers, perhaps a Rosary, and there would be an admonition from the priest to avoid sinful practices in the future. Confession just did not set well with me. In the confessional, Father Liebreich the pastor, once asked me if I would consider becoming a priest because he was convinced that I was basically a very good, sinless person. And I was. I said I would consider it. But that was the end of that. I had no interest in becoming a priest.

The second-in-command priest in our parish was a Luxembourger, Father Norman. He was big on anti-communism. His particular interest was the 1917 appearances of Our Lady of Fatima to three small Portuguese children. There they supposedly received three secrets including the prediction that the evil godless Russia would eventually reject communism and return to Christianity. Fair enough. I guess Russia has done that now.

One of Father Norman's pet beliefs was that the communists were out to destroy the USA, very much a popular belief in those days. When visiting our religion classes, he would ask the question, "What would our enemy do in our neighborhood that would destroy our way of life?" The answer was that one missile, fired at the commonwealth Edison generation plant just four blocks from our house, would knock out all of our electric power. This was an eye-opener to me and made all the kids very afraid. Curiously enough, with all the advanced systems available to our manufactured twenty first century enemies, taking out electric grids is one of the most talked about methods that an enemy could use to bring us to our knees.

4. MORE NOSTALGIA

My 7th birthday was on February 6, 1944. My gifts included several comic books and when I opened the wrappings and saw the covers, my body and mind vibrated. On one of the covers, in glossy color, was Superman flying in all his glory. He was full frontal, in tight pants and glorified crotch, and he wore a cape. Did my parents know that I was different? I cleverly took very short notice of the comic book covers, thanked them and placed the books aside until later, when I could dwell on that powerful, sexy image.

On my kitchen duty, hanging around in the kitchen, I learned at an early age how to make bacon and eggs. The bacon was cut in 1 inch pieces, browned and then I popped the eggs over them till cooked. I loved the security of the kitchen for other reasons as well. My mom was nearby me in her housecoat, and my trusty radio was on a little table next to the stove and in front of our huge south facing window. That room was my cocoon, my safe space.

My parents empowered me early to walk the one block to the corner market. A favorite item for me to buy was a loaf of Jewish rye bread. This was at the busy intersection of Elston, California and Belmont Avenues. George's Café was also there, and I could get my ice cream cones from George for seven cents.

Soon I was encouraged to go to another specialty store to buy smoked fish for our meatless Friday evening suppers. The fish store was uphill, a block away at the river, next to the Belmont Avenue Bridge. I needed to approach the shop by carefully stepping down old steep rickety wooden stairs to the river bank, where this tiny place was precariously perched. Meekly I gave the clerk my order, "Smoked fish please."

The Chelovich Pharmacy and the Fox Theater were two other popular businesses at the nearby, busy intersection. A tiny store that sold only tobacco was located in a round building that was smack dab in the middle of the small island in the middle of three streets. Another unusual and impressive building sat on another corner. It had colonnades and formally housed the Immel State Bank that went bust in the Great Depression. My family lost the money they had on deposit there when the bank failed in 1933. During my childhood, the building was used as a storage warehouse for nuts and bolts! For many years when we walked by, we saw nuts and the bolts stacked up behind the windows.

Bruno's Tavern was in an old dilapidated building at the corner, and it was my father's watering hole. He stopped by there at 4 PM after his shift ended at Western Electric. At Bruno's he could relax and enjoy a few beers with the neighborhood men. When I was four or five Dad would occasionally take me into the tavern, and I was fawned over by the men drinking there. I was a bit overwhelmed by the all-male scene. After this ritual Dad came home and almost immediately we had an early supper.

In the summer of 1944 my life was disrupted when grandpa dropped dead of a heart attack on the sidewalk in front of our flat on Belmont Avenue. This was bad timing for him and my grandma. Grandpa had just retired and planned to move from city life and spend full time in Delavan in the country. Fortunately, Roosevelt's new Social Security program gave my grandmother some small but needed income for the rest of her life.

I saw my mom cry for the first time when she got the news of his death. I was upset to see her unhappy. Grandpa was in an open casket at the funeral home and dutifully, I took my turn to kneel and to observe my mysterious dead grandpa for the last time. On an afternoon shortly after my grandfather's death, while listening to one of my radio serials, the program was interrupted by a news bulletin. "President Roosevelt has died." I took only a moment to realize that this was important, so I ran out the back door and down the stairs where I called to my mom, "President Roosevelt has died." "Don't make things up," she said. "It's true; I heard it on the radio." It was true. I felt vindicated.

We lived just one block away from the Fox Theater, a venue that had seen better times in the 1920s as a vaudeville house, and it now ran second-tier double feature movies. My parents gave me ten cents to attend the movies on weekends. I saw my first serials there. Because my attendance was sporadic, I would catch bits and pieces of these serials but never the full stories. In those early years, I saw lots of westerns. Cowboys and Indians, Tom Mix, Hop-a-long Cassidy, Gene Autry and Roy Rogers. On Saturdays I got to see the action serials along with the main movie. *Flash Gordon* and all the ill-fated characters in serials left me in suspense just as there was a crisis in the storyline. This was most frustrating because I never saw all the episodes and never got completion from these stories.

I was enthralled by *Pinocchio*. The moral of the story was clear to me. Never tell a lie. It was one of my father's rare pieces of advice to me, "never tell a lie." Dad's further explanation was that it was easier to remember the truth than it would be to tell lies and get caught with the difficulty of remembering them. Other than that Dad was definitely "lassez faire" in his outlook on life and in my upbringing. Another time Disney's *Dumbo* was showing at the Fox Theater and I was asked to take my younger brother Tommy along with me on a Saturday afternoon. He was five and I was seven. As the movie progressed there was a scary scene. A circus tent was burning and Dumbo had to jump down from a high platform into a hoop below. At that point my brother started screaming uncontrollably and I was forced to leave the theater and take him home. I don't think I ever saw the end of that movie. I was mad. This was one of the earliest incidents that gave me an uncomfortable resentment of Tommy.

My early visits to the movies were never about checking on the film's starting time. I paid my ten cents and walked in at any time convenient for me and the movie was already running. When the film started again I became aware of some familiar action and that is when I got up and left. Sometimes seeing the end first was a spoiler, other times the first part of the movie finally explained the meaning of the second half.

Many years later I realized why I had the privilege as a youngster of going to the movies so easily and often. It was most likely to finesse me out of our small flat so that my parents could have some privacy and some breathing space alone, and this was a way for them to have a few hours of intimate time together.

Riverview Amusement Park was a great way to experience a fantasy-land in the flesh. The park was close enough that we could see the tower of the parachute tower from our front windows. The parachutes ascended slowly to the top and then billowed out, and we would watch their quick decent to the ground. My mom and her siblings had the advantage of going to the park as youngsters in the 1920s. I am sure that the nearness of Riverview was important to my grandfather for the benefit of his four kids, and so he decided to purchase a home nearby. My mother revealed that she had been a Mardi Gras parade "extra" in her youth and told of riding on an elephant in the annual celebration.

My first trip to Riverview Park was with my grandpa and my cousin Kenny in the fall of 1943. It was an easy walk, and as we approached the grand, colorful gates, I trembled with anticipation. My cousin and I had a rush when we saw the fanciful buildings and the rides. Grandpa treated us to a picture in an arcade photo booth. We were so cute in our matching striped T shirts, squeezed together for our photo.

Rides that I liked were the parachutes, the roller coasters and the Shoot-The-Chutes. The parachutes gave that feeling of weightlessness for the few seconds after you hit the top. The "Bobs" was the fastest roller coaster and was thrilling when the cars whipped over the hills. It was claimed to be one of the most terrifying rides in the country. "The Shoot-The-Chutes," was a ride in an open boat, down a watery track that started from a high tower. At the bottom, we always got wet from the spray kicked up when the boat hit the water hard.

At age nine I was allowed to go to Riverview alone and I had a disturbing experience during my purchase of a ticket to a ride. I was confronted by a security man who started questioning me about how I got my money to pay for the ticket. The woman at the ticket booth told him that I had stolen money from my mother's purse. The guard let me go, but I was shook up and thought it unfair that I had been falsely accused. I often wondered whether the ticket lady made a mistake or was somehow hateful and vindictive to little boys.

At the park after World War II, I remember gobs of sailors walking around the midway and I was impressed with how they looked in their sexy uniforms. There was a mystique there, but I had no thoughts of what my feelings meant, or what I would actually do to act on them.

One memorable outing with my dad was when I was eight. He was a big Cubs fan and I often listened with him, to the games on the radio at home and in the car. Home runs were particularly exciting to me. The batter would hit the ball and the announcer would revel in saying "It's going way, way out and over the left field wall" for a homer. Andy Pafko was my favorite player. He played both center field and third base and he hailed from my dad's home state of Wisconsin. The first actual game I saw at Wrigley Field was with my father in 1946, a year after the Cubs won the National League Pennant. We took the Belmont Avenue bus, newly converted from streetcars, and got off at the railroad tracks that ran four blocks north to Wrigley Field. We "walked the tracks" as part of a ritual that my father followed when he was younger. Balancing on the rails I found surprisingly easy. As I entered the stadium I anticipated seeing a huge endless playing field of my radio imagination, but was introduced to the reality of its finite size. I was disappointed. The field that I imagined from listening to the games on the radio was far bigger, almost never-ending.

As a youngster, I was awed by two books we had in the house. They were essentially picture books, one commemorating the ocean liner the *Queen Mary,* and one about the 1933-34 Century of Progress, a world's fair that celebrated Chicago's first one hundred years as a city. The scale of the ocean liner and all the details about the cabins and its impressive appointments fascinated me. Same for the world's fair illustrations that highlighted all the colorful Art Deco buildings. These were special books that lit my fire for architecture, city planning, and ultimately real estate.

I started to explore the city on my own when I was ten years old. I took the bus to the Natural History museum and the Adler Planetarium, both located on the site of the 1933-34 Century of Progress exhibition. My friends and I also took the long bus ride to Hyde Park, on the far South Side, to explore the exhibits at the Rosenwald Museum of Science and Industry, which was built for Chicago's 1892 World's Fair. I loved that museum and its many interactive exhibits because it opened my mind to a whole fascinating world beyond my own.

The railroad fair of 1947 was another impressive event for Chicago- the railroad capital of the country in those days. The pageants, and the exciting dream trains with their elevated glass-domed cars, were touted as the future of travel. A few years later the airlines fulfilled this promise, and those 1947 dream liners became redundant. Strangely, I had never to that time ridden on a real railroad train, and to this day have taken trains only a few times in my life. The elevated train (the "L") in Chicago was of course the exception. I travelled the "L" thousands of times, because it was the most efficient public transportation in the city.

5. MY FAMILY & EARLY SOCIAL SITUATIONS

I hated the times that I was in the spotlight. In the first grade, with my classmate Jerry Schumacher, we had to memorize a little song for presentation on stage in the school basement. I was in a state of fear during the whole performance. A few years later, at my piano recital at nearby Brands Park Auditorium, I had the same fright. Well, at least I got applause after these tense performances, but I really preferred staying out of the limelight.

My earliest playmates were few. Other than my cousins, I played with a neighborhood girl, who seemed less intimidating than the boys. I really preferred my own company and had no particular competitiveness or interest in socializing with kids my age, or my adult relatives. I was very timid and felt inadequate and just did not know "what to say" either to start a conversation or to engage in a discussion. I was so fearful that when encountering a neighbor or a classmate on the street, I often crossed the street to avoid the encounters.

It was many years, before I had enough drive to start observing and understanding what was going on around me. Bit by bit my modest experiences would begin to add up, and make sense of the larger world out there.

Being an avid movie goer, I was mystified by the fact that the people on the screen always knew what to say. The fact that their lines were scripted did not occur to me. I was actually more mesmerized by the characters in my radio serials, probably because I could use my imagination and project the action as being bigger than life. I clearly preferred listening to the radio than going outside to play, even though my mother often encouraged me: "Why don't you go outside for some fresh air."

Part of my insecurity resulted from the nature of my family upbringing. It was very tight lipped in our household. I remember very little conversation. Germanic reservation no doubt! Certainly, nothing intellectual or momentous seemed to be happening in our home. My father did have a few conversations with my mother about financial affairs when I was present in the room, but I was told not to repeat the details because they were a private affair. The conversation, if any, around the dinner table concentrated on remarks about the food we were eating. My family did, however, have the will to give me and my brothers the advantage of some valuable middle class values even though we were definitely a blue-collar family with limited means.

I palled around with my three "boyfriends," but rarely or never with any of my school classmates. Those three were my only really good and close knit friends, and were my core buddies all through high school and college.

Andy Schumi was my closest friend. He never made me uncomfortable. He lived downstairs and he and I went through grade school, high school and college together. My cousin Ken was another close friend. He lived across the alley and we spent a lot of time together in the city and in Delavan. Jack was the third member of our group. He lived several blocks away in a big old house with his many brothers and sisters. They had a big peaked roof attic which was a neat retreat where we could play ping pong and shoot the breeze. Jack's sister Marilyn became one of the gang as we got older. All of us neighborhood kids played outside games together. We were a healthy, harmless group.

Chicago winters were cruel. My bedroom had no heat and my feet were always cold. As a small child coming down the back stairway I was faced with shoveled snow as high as I was. At age twelve I got my first job delivering newspapers in the neighborhood. I find it hard to believe that I delivered papers in zero-degree weather on snow and ice-slicked sidewalks. My scarf would be dutifully pulled across my face and I was further protected with ear muffs, heavy gloves, double socks, and galoshes.

From the eighth grade through high school in the early fifties, my boyfriends and I would meet in the basement storage area of our building. In cold weather, we would sit in front of the gas heater to keep warm. Inside Andy's apartment we played Canasta, the popular card game of the era. In the background the black and white television set would often be turned on to the political shenanigans of the anti-crime Kefauver hearings, and also to the rabidly anti-communist, witch hunting McCarthy hearings.

Outdoor games intimidated me. I reluctantly went along with plans to play softball in the local cinder lot when I could not suggest an alternative more to my liking. I hated being confronted with fly balls coming at me at high speed, which I was supposed to catch. I was afraid of injury. An old incident haunted me, and shaped my reaction to flying balls, ever since I was hit in the face in my grade school playground. Thereafter any ball coming my way was the enemy. Many decades later at the beach, a guy from Hamburg, Germany taught me an effective way to focus on the ball coming towards me, so that it would be easier to catch!

When I started my paper route in 1949 I was a skinny kid, and needed the help of my mother to hoist the newspapers into my basket at the front of my bike. The *Chicago Daily News* newspapers were delivered to our front hall. I rolled them on our kitchen table and pounded them so that they were tight and ready to throw. Then they were stuffed into a canvas bag and I started my route. Can you believe that I retained this job all through my high school years? It was my main source of spending money after my allowance was cut when my father lost his heavy wartime overtime hours. My paper route also gave me independence, and the opportunity to get out into the world. There I reluctantly met neighbors and strangers that helped me to break me out of my somewhat reclusive, comfortable cocoon at home.

6. TALES OF DELAVAN
– OUR WISCONSIN GETAWAY

In Delavan, my major friend was Jerry Grant. He lived two houses down and was two years younger than I. He lived at a house that was previously owned by my grandfather's brother, Uncle Tony, who owned it until 1950. Jerry had two older sisters, Gloria and Nancy. Gloria was a sensuous blond and Nancy a perky brunette. We all played games on summer days. Jerry was attuned to the country life so I tagged along with him and took up hiking and hunting sparrows with my BB gun. Jerry was a hot, good looking little guy and we kids often played games including trying to "pants" him. I played it cool and pretended that I had no ulterior interest in him. We never did get to see much of his butt or his privates but I certainly wanted to.

We kids had another favorite hike that took us up to the gravel pit, a partially mined hillside that had exposed rocks and sheer sides. It was a world unto itself and it rose above the flat lands of the "Delavan Highlands" where we lived. We felt like kings of the world up there. On those rugged slopes, we were masters of our private universe.

I had another friend in the country who my parents encouraged me to befriend. I was eleven years old. Jim was a black boy slightly younger than I who lived with his mother in the servants building up at the showcase horse farm up the road. "He needs someone to play with" they said. I met with Jim and we spent some good times together that summer. He was shy, a bit like me. I have always been impressed that my family had an open and fair view about relating to people that were different from us. It was a decent Christian thing. I took heed of it then and have felt the need throughout my life to find out more about people with different backgrounds.

Life in 1940s Delavan was Heaven. Grandpa had bought a cottage there in 1926, and it was just a bare shell at the time. Grandpa undoubtedly bought is so that he and his family could enjoy the country to balance a more cramped city life. The houses were marketed mainly to immigrant families in Chicago, during the prosperous decade of the 1920s. A fantastic story that I heard from my cousin Kathleen much later, was that a roving salesman one day, rang the family doorbell in Chicago and convinced my Grandfather to purchase the cottage on the installment plan! That shows me his openness to change that helped bring his family into the middle class.

I have always been impressed that grandpa took chances early in his life in America. I like to think that perhaps I exhibited some of that spunk later in life when I took some important plunges into the unknown worlds of real estate, sex and marijuana. After Grandpa died in 1944 Grandma spent a large part of the year full-time in the country. All her children and grandkids were welcome as regular visitors.

There were thirteen of us at the table when my cousins, aunts and uncles were together. All of us, except Grandma, slept in beds jammed up in an uninsulated attic that was only five feet high at its peak. There were just two small windows on either end. At times, the attic was a place of refuge for me, very mysterious, private, restful yet energizing. It was hotter than hell up there in the summer and sleeping in the heat was a challenge. One night I was sleeping alone and a wild rain storm came through. A period of intense thunder and lightning repeatedly rocked the house and I was convinced that it was the end of the world. I started to say my prayers. After a frighteningly long time the storm and thunder ceased. I would live on!

We kids had some wonderful evening romps in the attic beds, when the adults were not around. When I was visiting alone in the summer, I had the chance to do more exploration in the attic. The v-shaped roof line came down to the floor on both sides in a rather abrupt way. Grandma had rigged a cloth curtain that hid the last several feet that was used to store items out of sight. Grandpa had a hunting rifle back there and we were not to touch the gun. Only once or twice did I give it a little touch.

Until after World War II there were only four homes on our street. All the rest of the land lay undeveloped during the Great Depression. Therefore, we had large areas to explore that had open fields of high grasses, dandelions, patches of thistles and trees.

The Delavan Highlands development had planted fledgling poplar trees in the 1920s, which by that time had grown to an often-unstable height, especially in high winds. They sure dropped a lot of leaves in the fall. We hated the work needed to keep the lawns clear of the droppings. A magnificent maple tree grew just outside our rear porch. As kids, we reveled on its rope swing and climbed up into its strong branches.

We had a small rickety wooden pier nearby where the channel began, and that provided us water access to the lake. The channel was dug out in the 1920s as a marketing feature, to entice buyers to purchase the modest houses. Two gravel roads straddled the channel and two single lane bridges crossed it at intervals. We would take our wooden boat and row our way out to the lake, often through thick patches of waterlily pads and seaweed. On the way, we might dip for clams and watch for turtles. It took about fifteen minutes to go the full length of the channel. When we finally reached the open lake, we felt free. We would row over to our favorite swimming and sunning beaches. We could explore the far reaches around the shoreline. Around the lake were several other mysterious channels to explore, but there was always the chance that in the open lake, a change of weather would bring winds and currents onto our little rowboat party.

Another special treat was when I got to use my Uncle Art's red kayak. It sat two people and we had to learn how to handle the double ended oar and to avoid rocking the kayak which might cause us to capsize. Paddling back and forth was quite an exercise, and because the kayak was unstable, its shellacked canvas covering was vulnerable to tearing.

On holidays our two families would often build a fire on the ground in the back yard. Local logs were our fuel. We threw whole potatoes into the glowing ashes, covered them with coals and cooked them into delicious treats that had crispy, tasty skins. We broke off thin branches from the trees and stuck our wieners on the pointed ends. This allowed us to dangle the sausages over the fire until the sausages burst. Sometimes we would have a special treat of white Bratwursts, a country delicacy from my father's youth. We played croquet during the day, and at night we would play tag and hide and seek games. My favorite sport was badminton. We strung a net and would play against our cousins and our parents. I became very good at the game and frankly, it was the only sport that I ever really liked.

Summers alone with grandma were the best. Her cooking recipes were out of this world. I helped her in the kitchen to make fruit pies. I rolled dough, and dropped dumplings into boiling water. Her cooking was an eclectic mix reflecting the variety of ethnic groups that lived in villages in Galicia, at the outpost of the Austro-Hungarian Empire. These were country style recipes borrowed from the Poles, Jews, Hungarians, Gypsies, Germans, and Russians who lived in the area. Her recipes were almost always without meat. There were endless dumplings with names that her fellow Germans gave them such as "hallupsies"- Rice and chives wrapped in cabbage. "Perhays"-Cream cheese sealed in dough and boiled in water. "Hait Kennadles"-Little twisted doughs cooked in water. "Vuchtas"- Beautiful huge doughy balls, "Semilvava"-Old bread with egg cooked on stove top and served with butter and lemon, and a special dumpling with a hidden prune inside.

We would often drive to downtown Delavan, a historic, old fashioned town with a population of 5,000. There was a Main Street paved with bricks, and two-story buildings dating from the late 1890s. One department store that we patronized had a pneumatic tube that wound around the high ceilings, and that sucked sales invoices and cash up to the accounting office on the second floor.

The Delavan Theater anchored the business district at the far end of Main Street. Main Street continued on past large impressive residences as it became residential and tree-lined. Further on we came to St. Andrews Catholic Church where we faithfully attended Mass every Sunday. Visitors from the city swelled the congregation to standing room only in the heart of summer.

As a young teenager, I had sense of freedom when I was alone and biked the three miles into town. I invariably ended up at the town library. I looked forward to these visits where I could roam the racks and leaf through a myriad of magazines. I found that athletes and dancers were the best subjects, and a treat was to find pictures of men showing skin.

Many years later when I was in college I started to sleep in on Sundays, eventually deciding not to get up and go to Sunday Mass in town. With good grace my grandma understood, because Grandpa went to church only on the big holy days, consequently my growing laxity regarding church rules was nothing new in the family.

7. MY NEIGHBORHOOD IN CHICAGO

My family lived just one block from the Belmont Avenue Bridge. It had a substantial tower at one end that housed the bridge master. When he saw boats approaching that were too high to clear the bottom of the bridge he would activate the warning sounds and start lowering of the traffic barriers to warn the vehicle traffic on Belmont Avenue. After sixty seconds two parts of the bridge roadway would slowly begin to rise. All traffic had to stop when the bells sounded and the gates started to come down. It was exciting to watch the bridge roadway go up and the boats as they passed below. I often wondered what I would do if caught on the rising roadbed, and I even dreamed about it, and I saw myself hanging on for dear life.

During the war years, we often walked over to the bridge to watch the building of mine sweeping ships used in the war effort. The sweepers would sail out the Great Lakes and emerge from the St. Lawrence River in Canada for service in the Atlantic. The ceremonial launchings at the bridge brought large crowds to watch these exciting Champaign launches.

Our residential neighborhood was in a transition area, that was cheek and jowl with a motley group of factories. There were not many homes nearby and neighborhood children were few. I liked it that way because it allowed me to go about the neighborhood and not have to deal with lots of kids other than my three safe boyfriends. During the 1940s our neighborhood was mainly blue collar, but after the war many families who were in better financial shape immediately started to move out to more affluent neighborhoods.

Ours was a predominantly German and Irish neighborhood with smaller groups of Polish, Italian and Swedish families. There was a tiny but prominent group of Armenians who were refugees from the early twentieth century killings by the Turks. My first haircut was from Mr. Nicholich on California Avenue, who cut off my baby curls. Our neighborhood pharmacy was Chelovich. My favorite soda shop was George's, whose owners were also Armenians.

My grandparents sold our three-flat building in 1944 just before my grandfather's death in 1944 and just prior to their plans to retire in Delavan, Wisconsin. They sold the building to another Austrian, Anton Schumi, who was a friend of my grandfather, and who represented a shared old country connection. The selling price was $7,000. The sale was bad timing for my grandmother because massive inflation hit after the war and the value of the property tripled practically overnight when wartime price controls were removed.

The Schumis and their son Andy moved into the basement apartment while our family continued to live in the middle two-bedroom unit. Andy and I began our long-lasting friendship as soon as they moved in.

In 1947 the Schumis rented the vacant upper three-bedroom flat to the Strauss family who were refugees from Austria. The Strauss's had three children. Their son Eric was a year younger than I. As it turned out the Strausses were Jewish. I have often wondered whether the Schumis were expecting a Christian Austrian family. Eric and I on occasion would interact as both he and I had stamp collections, so we would trade stamps. One time when we were together outside he explained to me that "playing" was a waste of time and that he preferred to do something more "constructive." That word, that concept, hit me between the eyes. Only much later did I realize the connection and the very mature focus that Eric had at that early age. It was a kind of focus and understanding that was a long way off for me, and only after I had a lot of life experiences under my belt.

Across the street from our home were several empty lots. During the war, there were mountains of coal piled high fully visible from our front windows. It was coal that heated the homes in the area which until 1946 had mostly coal fired heating stoves. Kitty corner from us was the Bally manufacturing complex where they built pin ball machines. There was a huge explosion and fire in their factory in the mid-forties and many employees died who were trapped in the building. It was shocking to see the inferno from our front porch, where we could feel the heat from the fire.

We had a pickle factory nearby and we neighborhood kids would hang around, and to our delight we would sometimes be given a free pickle from the barrel by the barrel packers. Slightly farther to the southeast was a tanning factory and when the wind was right it would send foul smells our way. There also were the "clay hills" on the banks of the river. They were created from slag that had been dredged from the bottom of the river. This area was off limits to us. However once or twice I went over the fence with my friends to play there when my brother Tommy saw us and reported me to dad who thereupon, in the bathroom, gave me my one and only spanking. This was another of my annoyances with my brother Tommy, and I resented his snitching on me.

Our inner city Northwest Side neighborhood was very safe. No gangs. No ruffians. This suited me just fine. I was bullied only once near my house by an unknown boy who took me on a bike ride against my will. Occasionally our tight group of four boys would ride to other parks in nearby neighborhoods that were unfamiliar to us. On one occasion, as we played on the ball field, a stranger rode off on my bike. My friends were able to chase him and retrieve it for me. What a relief. I was definitely looked after by my neighborhood friends and my classmates because I was younger and smaller than they were. I was also quieter and they perceived that I needed their protection at times. They were right.

Hobbies throughout my childhood were often low-key interests that consumed me for a time. My weekly allowance and my paper route earnings allowed me to afford these extras.

I was intrigued by the ads in the rear of magazines that offered the possibility to assemble a magic trick collection and I took the bait. The ads promised learning the secrets of magic. However, once I acquired the tricks, I rarely had the confidence to learn how to perform them well enough to perform them for my family and friends,

I started assembling a stamp collection. Catalogs illustrated stamps from all over the world. I found that the United States issued commemorative stamps, that were attractive works of art, as well as lessons in history. I was intrigued and I learned a lot about countries through their stamps. The most interesting were Azerbaijan, Egypt, China, Iran, Germany, and Yugoslavia. I remember the stamps of Nazi Germany with the images of the German war machine. Some stamps had been over printed with new amounts as inflation took its toll on the country.

8. MUSIC IN MY LIFE – THE 1940s and 1950s

Of course we had a piano in the house. Every good working class family with an eye toward culture valued this instrument. My first recollection of a music recital was in the WWII years, when my uncle Art played Debussy's "Clair de Lune" for our huddled family in the upstairs flat. There was something dreamlike and melancholy about that scene, played by candlelight during a wartime blackout drill.

When I was ten my parents decided to upgrade my musical abilities, so I started piano lessons with our Irish neighbor Janet O'Neil. She lived across the alley along with her mother, father and brother. One day during my afternoon lesson at her house, there was a commotion in the living room adjacent to my lesson in progress. It was Tom, her very drunk brother, ranting and raving through the house. This was too much for me to handle and it shocked my very existence. I was quickly bundled off. Thereafter Janet came to my house to give me lessons.

That family upright piano was a gift to us from Grandma, and it was squeezed into our very small front reception area. It had a feature to play paper piano rolls that would control the keys to the play the songs of an earlier era. In the piano bench I found a copy of sheet music that my mother played when she was a young girl. The song was "Blumenlied," a very flowery Germanic tune. I loved it and learned it on my own. After suggesting to my Irish music teacher, and asking if I could play it at my concert she reluctantly agreed. Apparently, the Germanic nature of the song was not her first choice for me, probably because that music was still out of vogue and was generally frowned on, because of the immediate aftermath of the war.

At age twelve I got bored with the practicing that lessons required and got up enough nerve to tell my mother: "I am bored." It was a phrase I made up, thinking that it sounded profound and would express my frustration. It worked. That ended my piano lesson career but my love of music did not diminish.

In the late 1940s I would go with my mother downtown to the Oriental Theater or the Chicago Theater to see a movie and a live show. I remember the big orchestral sounds, and singers like Billy Eckstein. Then there were acrobatic groups, animal acts and comedy skits. It was very much like the fare that Ed. Sullivan featured on TV later on in the 1950s. I was specifically impressed/shocked? by a performance by Billy De Wolfe, a popular personality fresh from several Hollywood movies. He did his shopping-bag-mama routine in drag. I was entertained but also confused and a little embarrassed to see this. Perhaps it was a bit too close to one of my explorations when I had donned my mother's house dress in one experiment in front of the bathroom mirror. Billy De Wolf's stage bits and drag mannerism seemed a bit too effeminate for me, and there was that uncomfortable feeling that it might be a hint of who I was.

Our church choir at St. Francis was directed by Father Norman. We sang for Holy Day events in the rear choir loft. One Christmas Eve at midnight mass, after several weeks of rehearsing the classic "Silent Night" (in German no less), the children's' choir got its chance to shine. We proceeded to sing while Father Norman directed the choir. He had trained us to sing particularly soft the "Himlischer Rue" phrase. "sleep in heavenly peace," and we sang it just right. He was ecstatic. We were ecstatic that he was so pleased. This was one musical lesson among many that helped shape my future appreciation of vocal music and enhanced my love of singing.

Our family finally purchased a record player in 1949. One of the first records my mother bought was, strangely, a country and western song that apparently turned her on. It was George Morgan singing "Room Full of Roses." Very surprising because she was a city girl, but obviously the roses struck a note, perhaps reminding her of the pressed rose that I found in old book of hers that reminded her of a wonderful earlier experience. She also bought a recording of Ezio Pinza singing "Some Enchanted Evening" from the Broadway hit South Pacific. We kids made some fun by mimicking his drawn-out vowels and Italian accent.

9. SEXUAL AND SOCIAL AWAKENINGS – AN INTRODUCTION TO FETISHES

As a child, while I was in the bathtub, my father came in to relieve himself. He knew I saw his genitals and he proclaimed that his dick and his pubic hair was what I could look forward to. Around twelve or thirteen I started playing with myself in our bathtub and I had my first orgasm. That first one seemed to last forever and I got scared. Finally, the vibrations subsided and I knew what a wonderful sensation I could create for myself.

My only quasi-sexual experience previously was at age eight when playing "doctor" in the bottom flat with several neighborhood boys. We did not actually do much but look. One of the boys had an uncircumcised cock, the only one I ever saw until I was in high school. According to rumor in Chicago circles, the Jews and the Catholics were circumcised for religious and health reasons. Because of my early exposure to this demographic, there were few boys that I knew who were uncircumcised. Only later in my twenties did I meet more men who were uncircumcised. Over time I was I able to make an informed opinion on which alternative I preferred, although beauty and proportion were the final arbiters of my preferences. Other than an overnight's sleepover with a neighborhood boy at age fourteen, where we played with our dicks, I had no sexual contact with outsiders until age 16 when I started visiting the dressing rooms at the lakefront beach houses.

A more grown up hobby, but more of a sexual urge, at age thirteen, I started collecting 4x5 pictures of nearly naked men wearing posing straps. I became aware of these erotic pictures from the small ads I would see in magazines at the library or in other risqué magazines that I was able to obtain from small "disreputable" shops around the city. I sent away to Los Angeles and was mailed the pictures in plain brown wrappers. My mind went wild when I ogled the great bodies; men with their posing straps that outlined their sexual equipment. These pictures were hidden in my personal upper bureau drawer.

The photos were delivered to my home address and I needed to intercept the mailman before the rest of the family picked up the mail. The pictures provided me with ample means to fantasize about my newfound sexuality. There were some even more explicit pictures that I had read about where men's genitals were blacked out with black ink. A scratch off would provide a full all naked view. I never was able to find these, however, as most of the blacked-out pictures that I scratched did not reveal anything underneath but raw paper!

One of my refuges was the bathroom. Although there was no lock on the door, privacy was respected when the door was closed. When I was home alone it allowed me to explore the clothes in the hamper including my mother's house dresses. I did on a few occasions step into one and then added some lipstick to my lips! A T-shirt flowing around my head completed the picture. Quite a beauty!

About this time, I made a pact that I would be forever young. Not sure whether I made a pact with God or with the Devil to achieve it. Since that time, I have had no particular interest in dressing in women's clothes or wearing makeup even on Halloween. (Well I have done some glam Halloween dressups, complete with selected wild face paint. I'll call it "Punk," or fantasy. It's made for some sizzling Halloween times!)

My first formal sexual education came from Father Norman, our priest at St. Francis Xavier grade school. Boys in our seventh-grade class were gathered around a table, and our priest proceeded to discuss the "facts of life." He made an extra point of showing us a drawing of a penis and balls and proceeded to point out how terribly ugly the male genitals were. Well, I did not think so, but kept quiet of course. The drawing he showed us was a particularly ugly depiction, but I dismissed it knowing better. Future encounters would prove me right.

At about age thirteen I started to notice, while looking over the railing from the Belmont Avenue Bridge, floating rubber johnnies (condoms). This was before I knew exactly what they were for. Once I found out I became enthralled with their connection to male sex and I developed a fascination with them. Soon I would go fishing for them using tree twigs at leafy spots along the river banks where I could access the shore. There was also talk from my classmates about rubbers hanging from branches next to the Chicago and Northwestern railroad embankments. Presumably thrown out by passengers having sex inside the train?

My father was a switchboard tester at Western Electric and he would periodically bring home rubber "casings" that were somehow used in connection with his work. At one point, I realized that the casings were virtually identical to condoms, albeit with stronger rubber and big enough to get the biggest dick inside. I vaguely remember experimenting with one.

One early sexually charged situation was at my kitchen table at age thirteen. It happened while I was folding the *Chicago Daily News* and getting ready to make deliveries on my paper route. My mother approached from behind and dropped in front of me a sex manual book for young men. Nothing else was said. I felt strange, sort of having been found out!

This was extremely emotional for me, and obviously for her, because several weeks before, I had been confronted by my mother with a packet of those pictures of young men in posing straps. She said to me at that time "this is trash." In fact, I had been ordering 4x6 photos from AMG American Modelling Guild in Los Angeles for at least a year. Again, my operating plan was to intercept the mailman before the rest of the family saw the daily mail. It worked for a while, but, clearly my mom got hold of one of the mailings and opened up the envelope containing the questionable pictures. She did hand them over to me, however, and she realized it was time to deliver a "facts of life" booklet for me to read. Very embarrassing for me, but nothing more was said at the time. Apparently, my father was kept out of the loop regarding these first sexual situations.

On only one occasion did my father have any input into my sexual education, and that was through a relative and a close friend of the family. Dad asked him to bring up the subject. One day after a ride home from a family picnic, I listened quietly while this relative asked me if I liked girls and what my feelings were about all that. I nodded, but played dumb, listened and said very little. From that point on throughout my teens while living at home I played it very cool and low key.

10. A DEATH IN THE FAMILY

In the fall of 1950 my mother became ill. I remember my parents looking up the definition of "Carcinoma" in hushed tones. Mom went for removal of her breasts and she improved for a while but then her health went downhill in 1951 and in the spring of 1952 she passed away.

For months, she coughed and deteriorated, and rarely came out of my parent's bedroom. I hated hearing her coughing and covered my ears during the night. My father faithfully slept in the room with her. One very early morning I was awakened and heard a commotion with the voices of my Uncle Ed and my father. Hushed tones, saying that mom had expired. I hid, transfixed in my room. They removed her body so that we kids would not have to see her dead. I declined going to the wake. Being in the spotlight was too embarrassing for me.

Over time and much later I have revisited the probable mindset of my father at that time. My father lived a long life but my mother was not so lucky, passing away at 42 when I was 15. I never got to know her from an adult standpoint. In fact, my memories of her were not that vivid or complicated. She was always there for me but in a low key, well-meaning way.

My Uncle Art came over at once and consoled me with the thought that someday there would be a cure for cancer. He took me on a ride to his cousin's house and I still remember the long walk up a flight of stairs where he told her that my mother had died. I was to remain brave. Art was my mother's brother who remained unmarried until he was almost 50.

For a time, I thought he may have been gay. He was an intellectual of sorts and fostered anger, because the Great Depression had prevented him from attending the Illinois Institute of Technology to become an engineer.

After my mother's death, my grandma Ascherl became the effective mother in our family. We were lucky to have her. Life went on and grandma spent much time with me and my brothers, both in Chicago during the winter and in the summer in Delavan. After a few years, my father married Clara, my mother's sister, a conservative practical choice of his because he was concerned for us children.

Although these were upsetting events for me, none of these volatile situations caused me to dwell on them at the time and I moved on with my life. Yes, it seems cold and distant, but I had already plotted my eventual escape from my family life, and I remained focused on completing my education so I could move out and have my own life.

11. HIGH SCHOOL YEARS

It was a big shock to be faced with a new school, new classmates and new habits. Andy Schumi and I had discussed which Catholic high school would work best for us. We decided on St. Michael's Central High School in the old German neighborhood parish that my grandparents attended early in the century. It had an enrollment of 400 boys and 400 girls in separate wings. It seemed less overwhelming than DePaul High School, which was bigger, and to me more intimidating, and certainly nothing like Lane Tech a really big public high school just 1 mile from my home. As it turned out St. Michael's was a good choice. I had one of the best high school educations that I could have wished for.

Prior to enrollment we had to attend an entry interview. In the summer of 1950 my father went with me to meet with Brother John, the principal. I was nervous and guarded and quiet, but all went well and I was accepted as a student. The boy's school was run by the Marianists, known as the Brothers of Mary. They were a liberal secular group of brothers but they knew how to use discipline! I was a good student so I had no problem with any of the teachers during high school.

In the school complex the boys and girls were educated in separate sections of the building. The education classes were handled as two entirely independent schools. The girls were taught by the Sisters of Notre Dame. It was an interesting arrangement to have a partner school for girls in the adjacent wing of the same building. Apparently, this was a proper and practical approach for catholic schools at the time. We were separate, but equal. There were also two separate lunch rooms, one for the girls and one for the boys. Both could officially mingle for activities in the gym, such as for basketball games, school assemblies, and dances. I had no interest in the girls during these events and was artful but wary when these co-ed exercises took place.

On my first day in German class Brother Mueller said, "You have a very soft voice, do you sing?" I said "Yes, I have, in my church choir." He urged me at once to audition for the glee club and I wound up singing as a tenor for four years. I thought at the time that I should have been a baritone, but there was always a shortage of tenors so a tenor I became. The camaraderie among the glee club guys was great, and the musical techniques that I learned turned out to be valuable ones. Being in the glee club strengthened the appreciation of music that I have to this day.

I really enjoyed singing. It was good discipline. The group sang a lot of old musical chestnuts. "Stout Hearted Men" was one of my favorites. I can remember the words and sing it today. Of course we sang "Ave Maria" and all the usual holiday fare, and the military songs from operettas, especially the Germanic ones. We performed in the gym and had concerts several times each school year. One instance stands out, where my father, step-mother and grandmother attended. Afterwards they were introduced to Brother Mueller, and my grandmother and he exchanged conversation in German. I was proud and impressed at the connection.

A surprise for me came after my first test in German class. Brother Mueller apparently prided himself on shocking his first-year students with a test that was overwhelmingly hard. No one was more shocked than I, when I received a failing grade of 67%. I was used to only the highest marks in grade school and this was my first ever failing grade. I doubled down studying my German and I never had a low score again.

Brother John, the school principal, also taught history class. One of my most memorable lifelong lessons came from him. I can see him now in front of the blackboard. He wrote in large letters: "MODERATION," meaning in all things one does. This advice remains with me and has helped me stay grounded and helps keep my occasionally more excessive habits under control and in perspective.

All students were exposed to the basic Catholic rituals of the time, such as adhering to holy days of obligation, and attending other focused religious programs. There were religious parades on the first day of May. May Day. That day was co-opted by the Church as a counterbalance to the socialist celebration in vogue in the Soviet Union, where it had heavy political and anti-capitalist purposes.

All through high school I appeared to be the "good Catholic" kid. There was a contest that students could enter which was to be on a religious theme, so I submitted an entry on the meaning of the Blessed Virgin Mary. My article was published in our school paper. I knew how to go along with the game by being affable and quiet. I continued to bide my time.

As in grade school, I became friends with very few classmates. Those boys that I felt comfortable around, tended to be easy going and nonjudgmental. In addition to Andy there were two other boys I knew from grade school, Richard and Ed, who also attended St. Michael's High School. On one occasion the three of us were going home from school on the Elston Avenue streetcar when they shared an experience that they had in the summer of 1951. While vacationing in California they heard a new pianist in concert named Liberace, who was a showman sensation. They thought he was cool but definitely a "fairy." Believe it or not, this was the only time in my four years of high school that I heard anyone mention that term or any mention of homosexuals!

Both Andy and I were chosen to be the official scorekeepers for our two school basketball teams. Brother Gerhardt, the coach, chose Andy and me because we had the same address and he knew we could easily coordinate our schedules to attend all the games. Our school teams were called the Lights and the Heavies. Players were chosen by height. On the Heavies were the Helwig twins, who were gorgeous sandy blond gods, unlike almost anyone else in school. I definitely had sexual yearnings for them.

A secret thrilling foray was to go to the basketball team's dressing room after a game, where I had to be discreet, but was able to see the guys in jock straps and naked as they went to the showers. This was a vicarious pleasure for me. Dressing rooms became an obsession with me for a long time in future years.

12. A RISQUÉ TEENAGER

During my high school years I had the chance to explore my sexual side in various ways. I had the freedom to go almost anywhere in the city by public transportation. Several parks were within biking distance, and I found that I liked to check out the dressing rooms of neighborhood parks to catch a glimpse of hot older guys. Jock straps particularly interested me.

Summer in the city was a great time to go to the beaches along the lakefront. Exploring by myself, I would go to Lake Michigan beaches to work on my tan and to admire the young men. This was my opportunity to check on the dressing room action at North Avenue beach and the beaches at Montrose Avenue and Oak Street. It was there that I started meeting guys for sexual encounters.

These meetings, though relatively few, were transformational. They started around age 16, and took place when I did not have my school studies to occupy me, thus I had the leisure time to explore the gay world out there. These early encounters were not at all conversation oriented, but purely for the forbidden sensual thrill. This was new territory for me and in retrospect I was taking chances that could have given me STDs, or gotten me into trouble.

My very first rendezvous was with a man in his 30s who I met in the shallow water at North Avenue beach. I made a date with him to go to the Oriental Theater downtown. He made a point to tell me that he was Yugoslavian. The theater was showing a western film starring Jeff Chandler, but that was not the purpose of our afternoon. During the movie, with a raincoat over our laps, the guy masturbated me several times. My dick was sore after coming so much. A second tryst followed when he took me to an industrial building west of the river near downtown, where we had sex again. He became a bit aggressive and overbearing at that meeting and I chose to never see him again.

Another thrilling incident was when I made eye contact with an attractive man in his 20s who was sunning at North Avenue beach. I said to myself *get up the nerve to walk over to him and ask him to go home with me.* We took the Belmont Avenue bus to my home, never talking. After getting off the bus together I told him to wait until I went up the front steps alone to my flat and then to join me. The rest of the family was out of town in Delavan so I had the place to myself. My conquest came in and I told him to be quiet because the neighbors might hear. We went into my bedroom and we proceeded to have sex partially clothed. It was the first time I sucked a cock. It was so warm, and this is the way that I lost my virginity.

One other meeting stands out in my mind. I was seventeen and it was with a young guy who took me to his apartment at Grand Avenue and State Street. The subway stairs came up at that corner. He lived in an old brownstone that had seen better days, as had most of the buildings in that area at that time. We got into bed and at some point he asked me if I would like to "fuck." I thought about it for about three seconds and said "Yes," thinking that he must mean sticking his tongue into my mouth. I quickly found out what he really meant. He did sort of penetrate me but it hurt and we did not carry that any further. He loved having sex with me and said he wanted to take me to West Virginia where he was moving. This was a moment of passion and desire for both of us, but that obviously went nowhere. It was way too soon for me to be leaving home, although his adoration certainly intrigued me.

Still in High School, and having no compelling sexual interest in girls I still felt I had to pretend that I did. My school buddies Richard and Ed were dating heavily in high school. I am sure they were having discrete petting sessions and perhaps more. They invited me to join a small mixed group so that I might meet some girls. The girls they picked for me were usually overweight and unattractive. I was more interested in interacting with their girlfriends, than with the girls they set me up with. As far as I know Ed and Richard never suspected me of being gay because I was very careful to avoid the topic of dating, and they perceived me as quiet and socially insecure.

During those times, I had to be very careful when looking at other boys or to be seen looking at risqué magazines. There was a tiny store at the corner of Elston and North Avenues where I transferred from the streetcar to the bus., on the way to high school. The shop had male-oriented, provocative magazines in the window. I never went into that store, I was even afraid to be seen looking into their shop window lest someone see me and put two and two together.

At some point when I was still dating girls I felt the need to learn how to become more "with it" in social graces. I decided to become adept at dancing so I started taking dance lessons at Arthur Murray dance studios downtown. I occasionally practiced the new steps with my first girlfriend at home, in our living room, with the door closed for privacy.

One other heterosexual experience during high school was at my boyfriend Jack's home. His sister Rita began to hang out with us boys. We had a few parties in their third-floor attic during my senior year in high school and at one of those holiday house parties I kissed one of the girls, and we had body to body contact while dancing. As this was happening I was wondering whether I would get sexually excited—but I didn't.

My thoughts about my sexual preferences were definitely in flux during my teenage years. I clearly liked men, yet there was that need to fit in to the straight scene all around me. I certainly had no inclination to "come out of the closet." That was not even a scenario that anyone understood in those days, including me. All in all, I was able to balance two lives, one seemingly straight, and the other my secret life: Gay.

A cause for my great trepidation was the upcoming senior prom. I had to have a date, but I was gay. I had no romantic or sexual interest in girls but knew that I needed to fit in as straight. At a dance class at the school gym I plotted to make contact with a girl I could to talk with and invite to this big event. I gathered all my courage, forced myself to be aggressive and finally invited her to be my date. She was a freshman, but would do. She accepted. The duplicitous deed was done. I had carried off another diversionary act, and eventually had a good time at the prom, and I succeeded in allaying any suspicion that I might be gay. A group picture of all the participants at the prom was printed in the school paper and there I was in the front row with a big smile and looking as if I really belonged. Mission accomplished.

As my high school years progressed I busied myself with getting the best grades, excusing myself from most social situations and exploring my sexual side while generally keeping a low profile. I knew that it would be some time before I could be my own person; until I could start living my life without the guarded limits that my world demanded. I would essentially be trapped for some time to come, in the conventions and expectations of the people in my daily life.

Hello to Rob

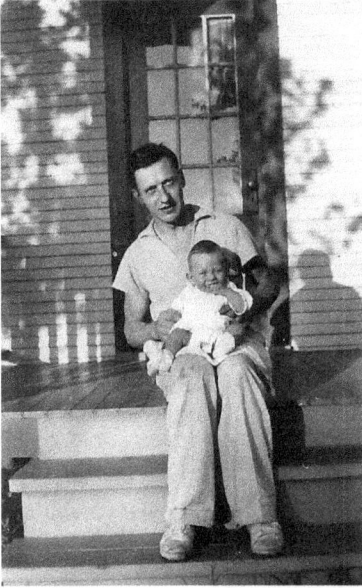

Dad and me in Delavan, Wisconsin.

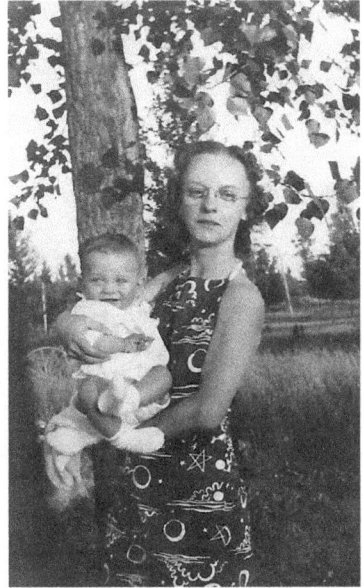

Mom and me.

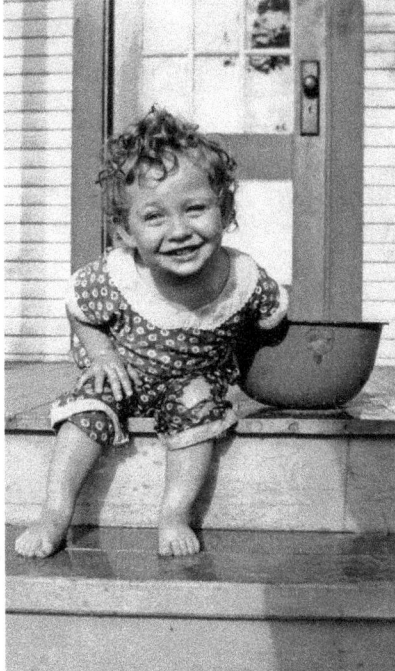

Hamming it up. Haircut next month.

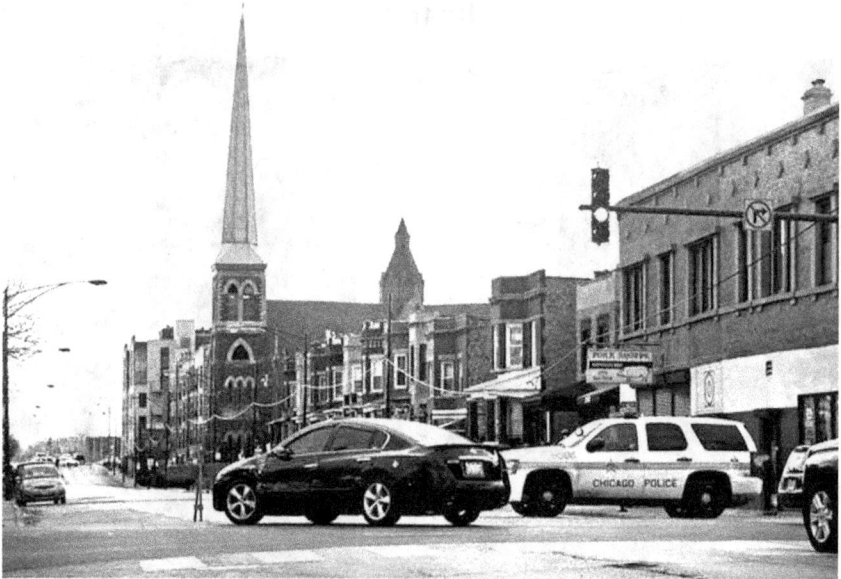

Concordia Lutheran and my Belmont Avenue block in Chicago.

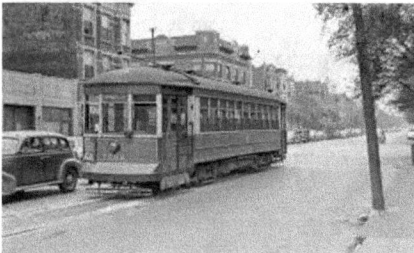

Belmont Avenue streetcars ran
outside our house until 1945.

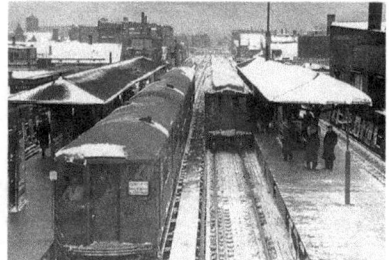

Belmont Avenue "L" station.
My frequent transfer point.

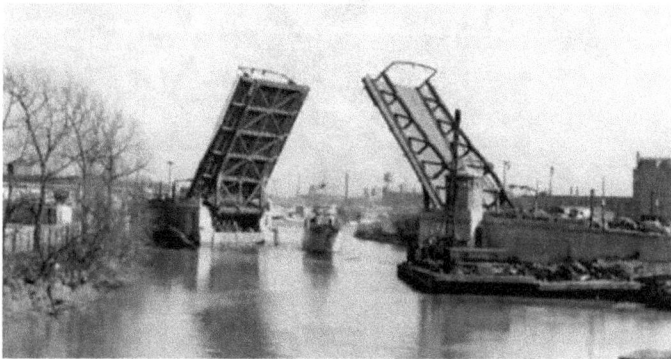

Belmont Avenue Bridge.
Site of fish store and mine sweeper launches.

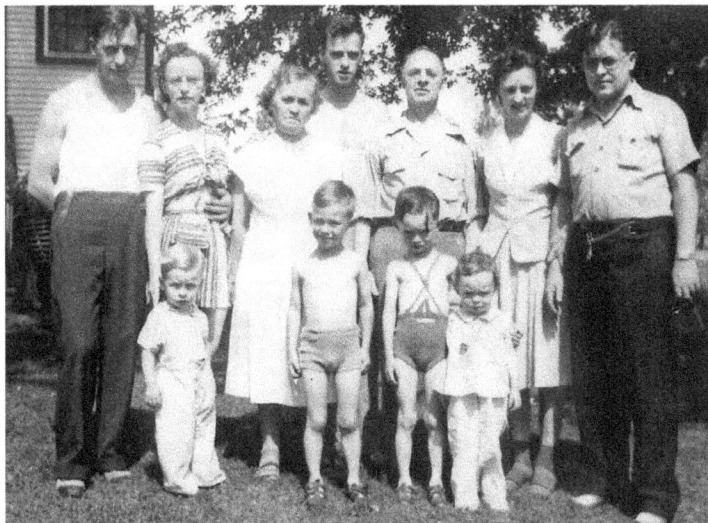

The Delavan clan enjoying grandparents' summer home, 1942.
I am the shirtless one.

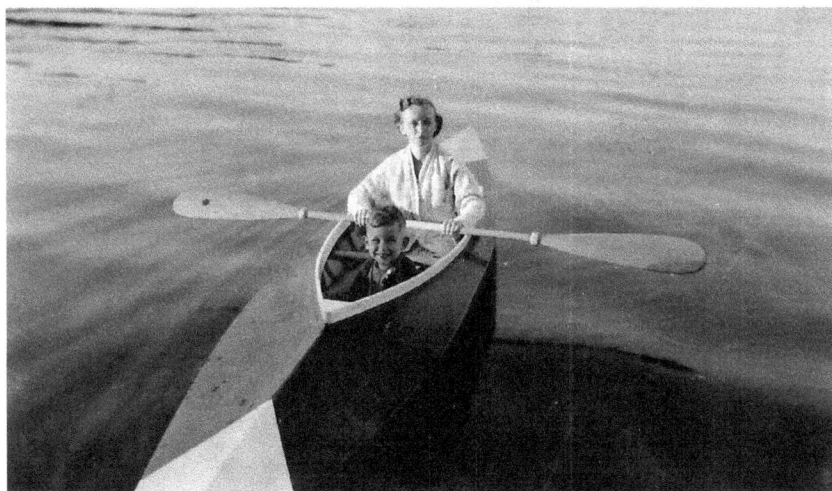

A serene moment with my Mother, 1940s.

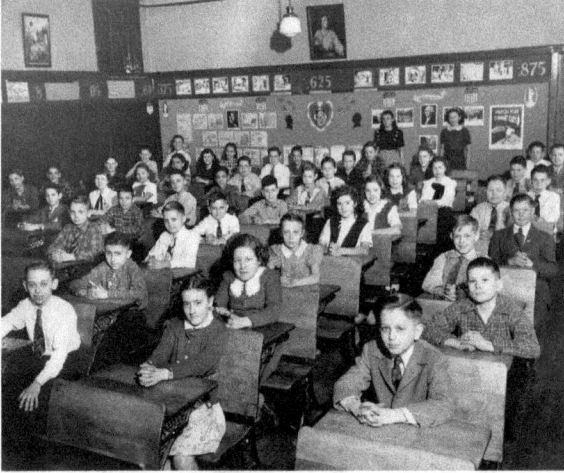

Sixth grade class. I am front row, left.
Always the shortest in my class.

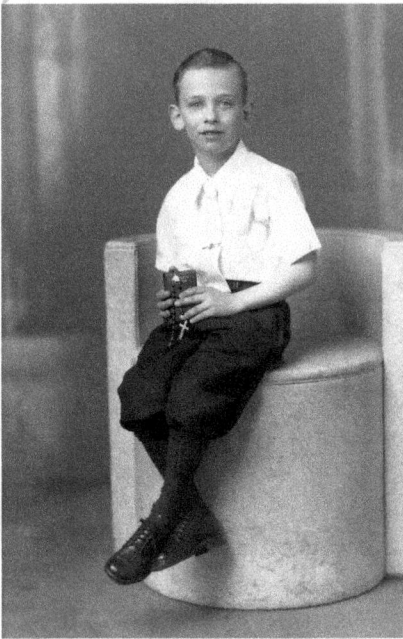

The "Pair-O-Chutes"
at Riverview Park.
Visible from
our front window.

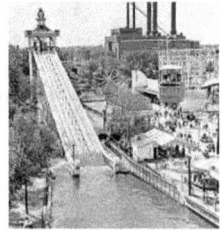

"Shoot-the-Chutes"
at Riverview.
Edison Power Plant
in background.

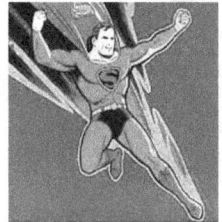

My first Holy Communion photo—a perfect boy.
I missed the ceremony first time around (fair warning!).

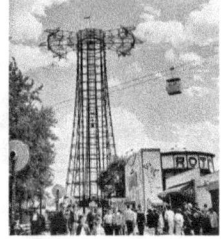

Superman surprises me
on my seventh birthday.
Have I been
discovered?

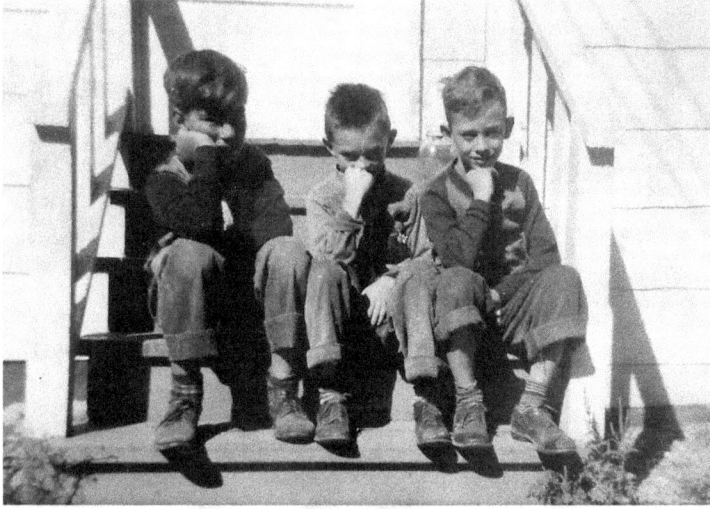

Three boyfriends in Delavan, 1946. Johnny, Kenny, and Bobby.

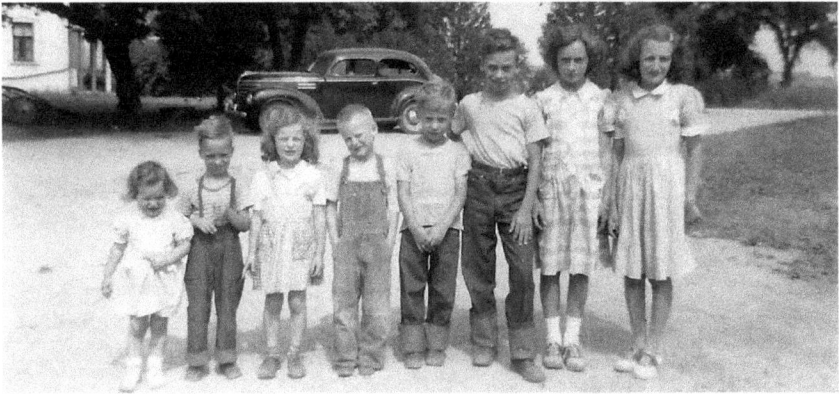

Country Cousins on Tackes homestead farm, 1948. Our '39 Plymouth in back.

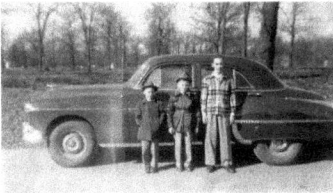

Our new 1950 Oldsmobile.
Dad finally felt safe with four doors.

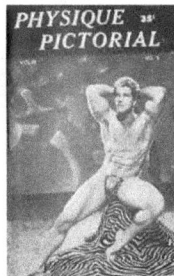

"Forbidden Fruit"
1950.

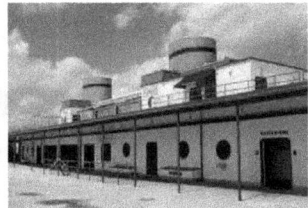

North Avenue Beach dressing
rooms. Site of clandestine
meetings.

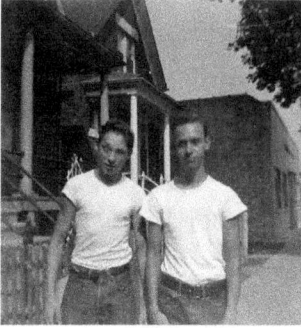

Toughies, 1952.

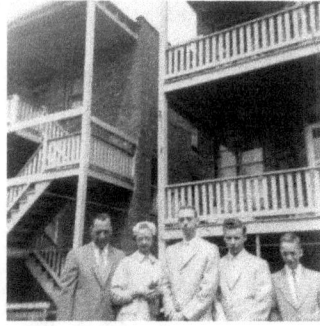

Typical backyard photo, 1955.

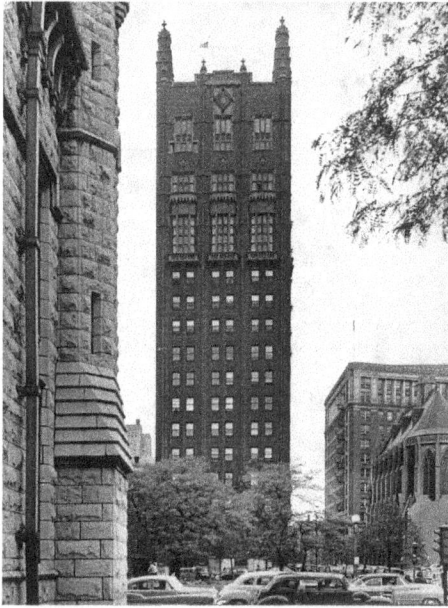

Lewis Towers, Loyola University Business School, 1954-58

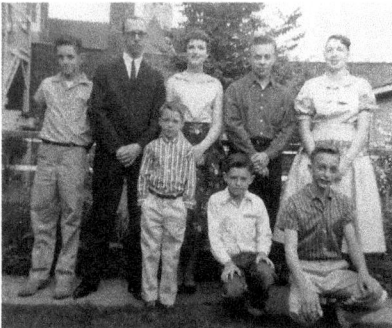

1958 B.Sc. graduation from Loyola,

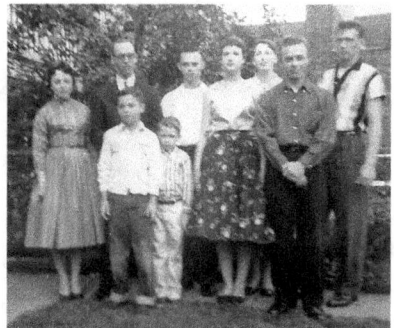

with my Chicago cousins.

Hello to Evanston

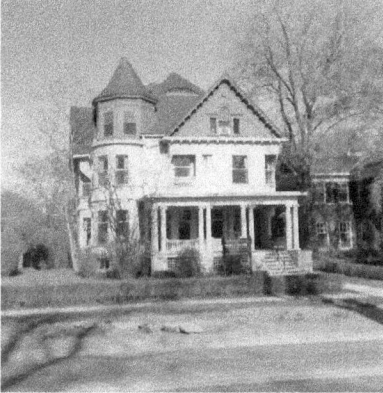

Third floor garret shared with
roommate Bob. Red velvet furniture
in living room.

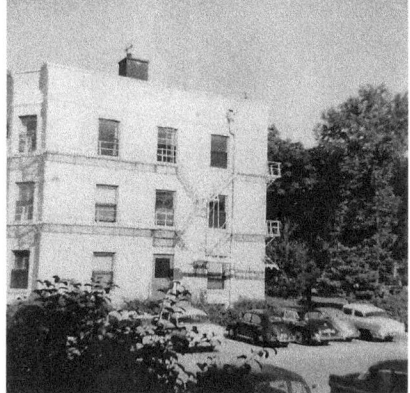

Meeting place. First date with Denis
at NU Music Annex.

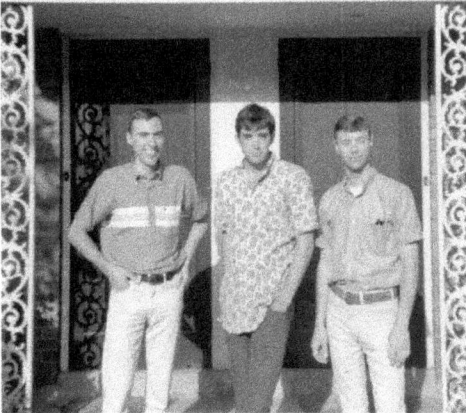

Denis, Paul, and Rob
in front of our townhouse.

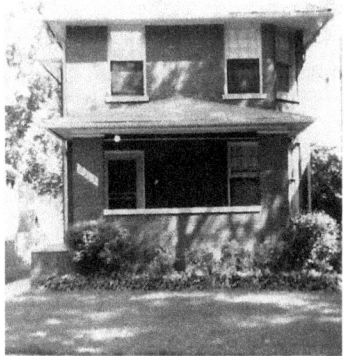

Our Evanston
investment property.

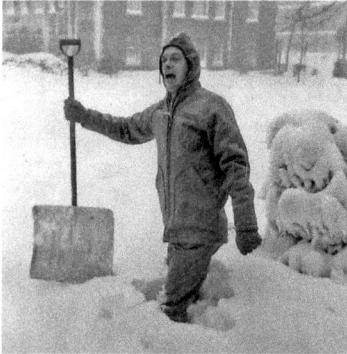

1967 Evanston blizzard.

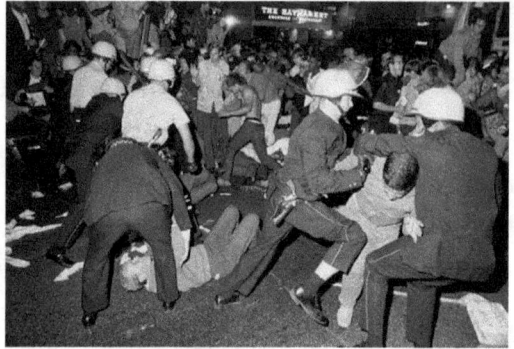

1968 Chicago convention riot.
I was caught in a mace attack.

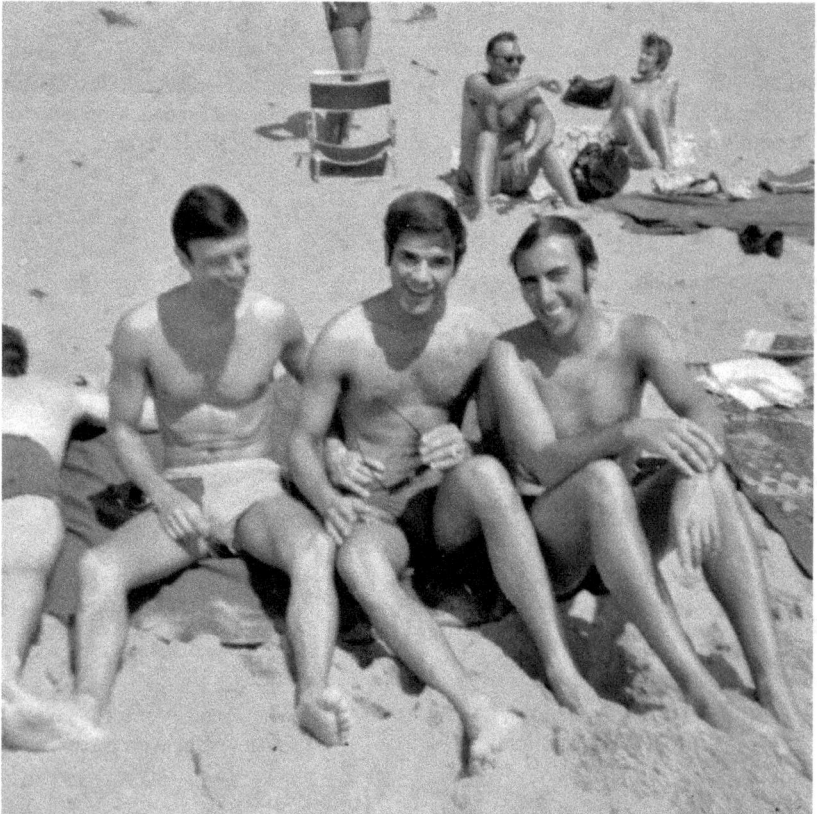

Late 60s Provincetown trio.
With Dan who later acclimated me to San Francisco.

13. UNIVERSITY YEARS

In my senior year in high school a big challenge presented itself, when I was faced with deciding where I would go to college. As a result of my high grades, I had won a full four-year scholarship that would pay my way to a catholic Marianist college in San Antonio, Texas. However, I did not want to leave home and abandon the big city with its abundance of opportunities to continue my gay explorations. I knew the winter weather would be kinder in Texas but decided to play it safe. I turned down that four-year scholarship and instead accepted two $500 scholarship awards, which were enough to pay for my first two years at Loyola University Business School. I chose an accounting major because that was a profession that I could visualize for myself, given my naïve ideas about what other careers might be like. This was a real toss of the coin event that affected the rest of my life.

Staying put in Chicago I could continue to live at home, work part-time jobs, and have time to ponder my future in familiar surroundings but it also presented me with challenges, but I saw them through.

Here is what living at home while attending college was like. The lack of space in our tiny flat was a problem. In order to accomplish my studying, thinking and typing I needed to hole myself up in the bedroom. The sound from the TV in the living room was annoying to me. My bedroom had no heat, and in the winter and I had to be really creative to stay comfortable. My 1920s Underwood typewriter sat on my super small desk, all this cheek and Jowell against the wall in front of one huge window. This meant that the cold Chicago winter temperatures and frigid winds were right outside, inches in front of me, and happy to seep through and freeze me. I often had to wear a pair of heavily insulated boots to guard against cold toes. I purchased an inexpensive rudimentary space heater that helped warm my feet. Sometimes it blew the house fuses. Those were the monk-like conditions that I put up with when I studied and typed out my important papers for school.

To enjoy some privacy and warmth I spent lots of time studying and doing research at the main Chicago library on Michigan Avenue. Their great room was warm, quiet, and forgiving, almost sacred.

I was a study wonk all four years in college. There was little interaction with my family outside of my occasionally joining them to watch television. Dinners were always at 5:15 PM. Family conversation was never about much, certainly nothing controversial or intellectual. My father loved it when we had meat for dinner, which we could only occasionally afford. Having been brought up on a farm in Wisconsin, Dad was no doubt remembering the steak and sausages that he had all the time and that often came directly from the animals on the homestead. After dinner, I usually retreated to the bedroom to resume my studies. The family went to bed early for dad's next 5 AM awakening to go to work.

During my time in high school and college grandma Ascherl acted as a mother to me and my brothers. She was a wonderful person and very kind to us. Jerry, my youngest brother, was only seven years old when mother died. Grandma took responsibility for Jerry and spent many long periods with him in Delavan, Wisconsin during the summer. For that reason, I remember very little of him because I was immersed in my life, my schooling and my part time jobs.

After my mother's death in 1952, Dad felt the need to provide a new mother to the family. Eventually he decided to play it safe and announced that my mother's sister Clara would become his wife. Clara was the eldest of four children. During my young years, she travelled the world at positions with the federal government. I remembered only a framed photograph she sent home in the early forties, where she displayed a trendy, very short hair style. My grandmother did not like that look! After the war and the death of my grandfather, Clara decided to live with my grandmother full time in the cottage in Delavan. After one winter in that uninsulated house they realized that it was too cruel to spend winters in the bitter Wisconsin climate, which was even worse than our Chicago winters.

My dad married Clara at St. Francis Xavier church after having been vetted by the Catholic Church hierarchy, all because Dad was marrying his first wife's sister. Apparently, this was a medieval taboo. I was best man. This *was* weird!

Living at home with a new mother was a challenge for me. The shit hit the fan several times and we both saw the need to adjust. For example, I was shocked when she announced that she would no longer be ironing my shirts. Only later on upon reflection did I understand the time and trouble it was for her to do that kind of drudgery. One other run-in with her occurred when I was in the living room listening to my new recording of the Poulenc Organ Concerto. The piece had several exciting, ominous, low sequences where the Organ went wild. She came running into the living room and said "What is that?" in disgust. I yelled back "This is decent classical music." Our relationship was never the same after that. We became distant and just did not have the ability to ever work it out.

Back to my studies. Loyola's Business School was based in their downtown campus at Lewis Towers, a 1920s residential high-rise that was converted to offices and classrooms for the students and faculty. Its location was directly across the street from the historic Chicago water tower on Michigan Avenue. Right around the corner was Rush Street, Chicago's main nightclub district. Also nearby were Hugh Hefner's offices, where he had just started his fledgling *Playboy* magazine and eventual empire. My easy commute to college was on the Belmont Avenue bus to the "L" at Halsted Street. Eventually the "L" cars went underground and continued as the subway to the Chicago Avenue station just a block away from school.

Part-time jobs during my college years paid for my expenses. They allowed me to save enough to pay the tuition for my Junior and Senior years. Loyola helped me find a job at Montgomery Ward ("Monkey Wards") which had their main corporate and warehousing offices on Chicago Avenue, conveniently close to Loyola. After my classes I would hop on the Chicago Avenue bus and could be at my Montgomery Ward job in minutes. There I did auditing and reviewing of operational paperwork sent in by their stores throughout the country. Boring as hell, but it was a stable source of income.

My studies and my desire to get top grades continued along the same lines as in high school and I continued to hide my gayness. What major concepts did I learn in collage? Here are some moments at Loyola that stand out in my memory.

My very first class was *Statistics 101*. We were assigned to read *How to lie with Statistics*, and from that exposure I became forever aware of the glories and the pitfalls of using figures, charts and percentages. To this day, I can see the potential defects in many presentations that involve statistical comparisons.

Professor Mogulnitsky, who was a white Russian escapee from the revolution, taught Economic Geography. He made a major point that I have incorporated into my life, He said that long after the detailia of his course were forgotten, the most important thing that we could do throughout our lives was to "stay current." He recommended reading as many pertinent magazines on any subject that interested us. He promised that it would keep our minds agile and in touch with reality. He was right. For years I subscribed to magazines like *The Atlantic Monthly*, *Harpers*, and *The National Geographic*. Much later I came to realize the benefits of newspapers like the New York *Times*, and later on the internet would fuel my insatiable interest in staying current and to entertain new ideas.

In addition to business courses, we had courses in Logic and Philosophy, which had a lasting effect on my future thinking. The benefit of that exposure has helped me to see the defects of many crazy emotional ideas that others take seriously as gospel. At the time, I understood only part of those high philosophical concepts, but the formulas and disciplines in those classes stuck with me. If it doesn't make logical sense, then maybe it is BS. Logical thought, as I came to believe, is the masterful incorporation into the human dialogue of an important grounding element. It is an element that is often missing in discourse, especially when ideology is introduced into the mix.

One other awakening during my college years was of the world outside the business realm. I signed up for an after-hours informal group that met with the professor of our history class. We discussed music and film and were introduced to obscure artists like Geraldine Farrar, an early 20th century opera singer. We were also encouraged to explore the newest wave of foreign films that were being shown at Art theaters in Chicago. Thus I ventured down to the Auditorium Theater on South Michigan Avenue and saw *Diabolique*, a French film with an awesome terror scene. I made my first visits to the suburban North Shore's Ravinia Park to hear the Chicago Symphony play in their idyllic, sophisticated setting.

In 1957, during my last summer at home, I purchased a 1953 Studebaker coupe. It was a beauty, low slung and with Italian styling. The price was $600, which I did not have, but I was able to get my dad to pitch in half, which amounted to my graduation present. It turned out that the car's engine was a dud and it burned lots of oil. The mobility that my Studebaker gave me was a godsend, however. I could now drive to Delavan on my own. No more public transportation in Chicago, so I could drive to my Lewis Towers classes downtown, park nearby, feed the parking meter and then whip off to my Montgomery Ward job after class. My car made it easy to get to the newly discovered "Belmont Avenue Rocks" in the summer, where I had some of my first encounters with gay men, and where we all were out of the closet for a brief time, in our own special world.

Further masquerades of dating girls continued during this time. There was Mary Margaret, a proper catholic girl and after dating her for several months I gave her my class ring. Our breaking up was as traumatic as my resigning from a job. It always pained me to separate, and say that I was moving on. My relationship with another more savvy girlfriend during my senior year in college turned out to be short and mercurial. I travelled to Grinnell College in the Tri-Cities in Iowa to join her for a social weekend. This was my first long trip in my Studebaker. I arrived on campus but she hardly paid attention to me. I think she had me pegged for gay. This was the last time I had to pretend to be straight and interested in women. I would move on exclusively to men after graduation, although I still remained in the closet as far as the general outside world was concerned.

As my final year in college approached I become more restless about my future away from home. But I was also excited and looking forward to a brand new life. There was one last dilemma about whether I would embrace the Catholic Church. After attending an obligatory heavy religious retreat, I made my one and only "true" confession where I admitted my gay acts to a priest. This was terrifying! However, the gay option was becoming clearer, and just before graduation I chose to leave Catholicism behind. I now had my Bachelors of Science degree in Accounting and was ready to pursue a new life.

14. AN EMBARRASSING MOMENT

In my junior year at college I joined a gym to start getting myself into more attractive, muscular shape. I was small boned, short and thin, so this was my way to become more attractive to other men. The gym I joined was located downtown, with a second location on the far North side, just south of Evanston. I got into a conversation with several of the straight guys at the downtown location who mentioned stag parties that took place regularly. The parties were on the far South Side and included sex shows. I discovered that in Cuba they were called *"exhibiciós."* I was intrigued, so I took the "L" to an evening party in a mixed neighborhood that was in a black transition area. The gathering was in an apartment building and the admission was $2.00 with beer for sale on the premises. A crowd of around 40 people was jammed into the flat and everyone was expecting the action to start soon, and it did. A Caucasian couple stepped out, a guy with red hair, and a buxom woman, and they proceeded to have intercourse on the floor in front of the panting audience. Sex for pay was available to any of the attendees who cared to follow up later. I was too vain to wear my glasses so in the darkened room I crawled closer to get a look at the penetration that was taking place. I had no qualms and fixated raptly on the sturdy man fucking the woman. I was so turned on that later that night after I returned home, I spent all night in a half-awake state, and had the most number of incredible and intense orgasms while recalling that guy fucking the girl.

Some weeks later I attended another party at the same location and while the crowd was waiting for the action to begin there were delays, and more delays. Suddenly one guy sitting next to me on the couch got up along with several other men in the apartment, and said "everyone stay still where you are, this is a raid." Ohhh. The police had not been paid off enough. The owners were charging for alcohol without a permit, and horrors, devious sex was taking place. Well, up pulled the paddy wagons and we were all herded in through the rear doors and taken to the precinct police station and booked for being inmates in a disorderly house. Probably forty or so people were arrested. Eight to Ten of us were put in a cell together, it was about ten PM, and I was miles from my Northwest Side home. My parents had no idea where I went that night. Quite a dilemma.

In the cell, we had one hole in the floor which was our toilet. I was terrifically pee shy and suffered from a bloated bladder for a long time until the rest of the party dozed off and I could urinate. All night long other miscreants were booked into the jail and the cells were full of drunk, unruly people. There was screaming and swearing and tin cans were being run across the bars. In other words, general hellish mayhem. I did not sleep.

In the morning, the jail staff served us baloney sandwiches. Gradually the group was allowed to leave the jail, but on a very slow case by case basis. Apparently, some individuals were able to reach attorneys who started the release process. I thought I would be released soon after seeing person after person being let out from our cells. At six PM that evening I was still in the cell with only one other person. When he was about to be released I panicked. I asked him to please call my home number to inform my family where I was, and to come down to bail me out. The thought of spending another night in the cell was frightening as hell. Several hours later the cell door was opened and I was released. My uncle Ed had driven down along with my stepmother Clara. I said to them "get me out of here." The drive back to the North Side was eerily silent. I explained that it was a Stag Party that had been raided. They understood. I was terribly embarrassed, but at least the party was a straight event so there was no hint that I was gay. As was the case regarding other personal and emotional situations in my family, this incident was never mentioned again. I am sure that my father was spared the knowledge that this had happened, for he was at work and did not participate in my spring from jail. The local South Side neighborhood newspaper printed an account of the raid with all our names. (My name was, unfortunately spelled correctly!). I rationalized that no one from my family would see the article, because the event took place way on the other side of the City. Apparently that was true, so it saved me and my family from further embarrassment.

PART TWO

BREAKING FREE
Wild Times

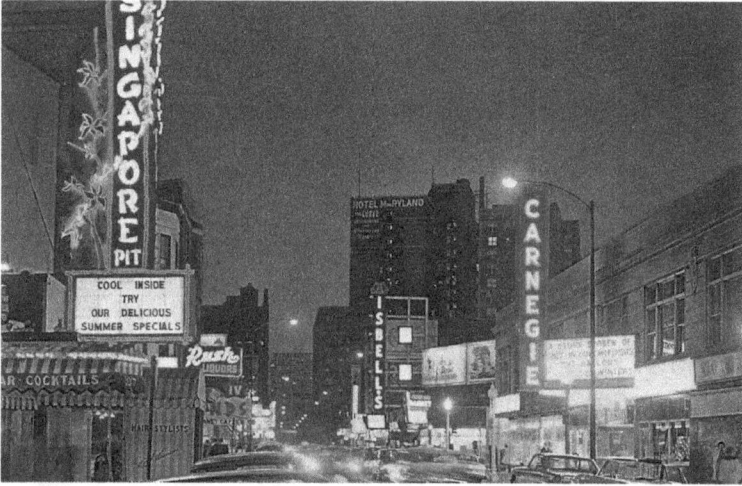

Rush Street. My first legal drink.

15. MY FIRST GAY AFFAIR

An important event took place my junior year in College. It was at the fiftieth wedding anniversary for my uncle Tony and aunt Lizzy.

I was introduced to Arthur, a handsome guy nine years my senior who was a student at the Art Institute of Chicago. Upon being introduced to him something instantly registered with me, and a special chord was struck. We hit it off and he invited me to an after party at his aunt's home in Park Ridge. Upon arriving, the daiquiris were flowing freely and the conversation was a lot more adult than I was used to. All in all, an eye opener. Arthur offered to give me a ride home sometime around 3AM on that blistery cold night. We were both quite inebriated. He drove, and we slid out of control several times on the glistening deserted city streets. Along the way, we started to embrace. He pulled the car over to stop on a residential side street where we got out and made out as best we could in our alcohol-induced condition. Nothing happened to completion but the ground was laid for some further more proper social meetings with him.

Over the next few months I finally summoned my nerve to call him, which I did, and he invited me to his flat for lunch. His apartment was in Old Town, which at that time was a trendy, artsy area just north of the downtown. Arthur had a roommate, Mickey, who had a job in advertising. It was gradually dawning on me that He and Art were lovers, a new concept for me which I had not given any thought to yet. At the time, the idea of a gay, long term relationship was not in my mind, in my simplistic and rather narrow experience. It was a wonderful lunch. Conversation was guarded but pleasant. There was something terribly attractive about Art's lifestyle and I wanted to explore it, and him, more in the coming months.

Soon thereafter I asked him out for a drink. He suggested a dark, atmospheric place on Rush Street and we proceeded to down two or three strong Daiquiris. I had eaten some white bread before our meeting so that I could keep up with Arthur who I gathered was an accomplished drinker. One thing led to another and we checked in to the Belmont Hotel on Sheridan Road at the lake front as uncle and nephew. We both were very high from the hard liquor and we wound up in bed. We went through a number of furtive motions trying to cum but we didn't succeed. This was my first experience spending the night with someone I knew.

Another early experience was the day of my 21st birthday. I went out to celebrate with one of the fellows I worked with at Montgomery Ward. We walked from Lewis Towers to a bar a few blocks away on Rush Street. After a few drinks, we decided to go to his place where I proceeded to sleep the night with him on a very narrow bed. I was petrified to do anything sexual. In my naiveté, I was not really sure he was gay. So I played it safe. We wound up sleeping very close together but there were no sexual moves made by me or by him. A long time later, years perhaps, I recalled this experience as somewhat juvenile and immature, especially and ironically because my co-worker's last name was Bedgood. Nothing more ever came of this incident and we did not talk about it at work or ever again.

During the spring of 1958 I was meeting other gay men at the Belmont Rocks and other places around town. The Belmont Rocks was a notorious gay area for sunning right on the lake.

Another attraction was a gay bathhouse in the basement of the Lincoln Hotel. It was a very mysterious and forbidden new experience the first time I went. A cute blond that I met at the Belmont Rocks had invited me. The steam room was steamy, slippery, but dreamily sexy. It was, it turns out, also a great place to pick up a Sexually Transmitted Disease. That reality set in when I soon caught my first case of "crabs." I discovered that there was a preparation I could buy at the pharmacy that would get rid of them. Prior to that I thought I would have to pick them off individually or shave them off. I was still quite naïve in the scheme of things gay.

My downtown gym was no longer appealing to me so I switched to the Howard Street branch on the far North Side at the border with Evanston. At the gym I met Bob, who lived in Evanston, and who intrigued me because he was southern, and a laid-back conservative. One day in the shower room we started a conversation and I probed a bit about his social life, thinking that he might be gay. After a bit of verbal fun back and forth in the shower area I found out that he was going to go to a bar that weekend down in the city. Without losing a beat I said "is it Sam's Place?" His jaw dropped and he said yes, and would I like to go. I had no idea that such a bar existed. I pulled "Sam's Place" out of some unknown recess of my mind and I almost said "Pete's Place," but thought that Sam's was a more likely generic name to use.

Sam's was one of the most notorious gay bars in Chicago. It was a nationally known institution on the near North Side of Chicago, on Clark Street near Grand Avenue. Many gay celebrities dropped in from time to time to slum a bit. Within days I went with Bob to Sam's for my very first gay bar experience. Walking into this dive was exhilarating, frightening, educating. Every imaginable type of person was in that bar. Sleazeballs, drag queens, rough and tumble men, old and young, all seething and pulsating with sexual energy. I soon returned to Sam's by myself to reinforce the powerful draw that this kind of place would have for me in the future.

16. ON THE CUSP OF A NEW LIFE

During my last year of college I was enjoying this newfound social world, and, as a result of my exploits, my senior year grades suffered. My '53 Studebaker provided me with cherished mobility. At school, my A's turned to B's but I was less concerned than ever about my grades because I was really enjoying my new lifestyle, and more importantly, the rest of rest of my life was finally coming into sharper focus.

My attention was shifting to where I would move after I left my cramped, limiting life at home. I had visited Evanston, a solid, old line suburb just North of Chicago on the "North Shore." My uncle Art often took me on trips there throughout my childhood. It always seemed like another world and it would prove to be just that.

I visited my southern friend Bob in Evanston to get a further feel for what I suspected was to be my new home. Just before my graduation he and I went to the park just south of Northwestern University campus that had huge breakwater boulders lining the shore of the lake. I remember that spring day in 1958 when I went gaily tripping the light fantastic on these rocks with Bob, and saying out loud to him "what a wonderful time to be alive." He agreed. I knew then that this was to be my new heaven.

17. GRADUATION AND SEPARATION

My Loyola University class of 1958 matriculated in late May at a movie palace on Devon Avenue just south of the main campus. Within a few weeks, I made plans to move to Evanston and informed my father the very day that I was packing to move out. Dad expressed some sort of feeble hurt and surprise, but that was it. I loaded a wooden fruit crate with my books plus a bunch of my clothing, loaded them into my Studebaker and drove north to my new life.

My first home was an attic room at 1931 Orrington Avenue. It was a huge fantastic Victorian home just 1 block off Northwestern University campus, and one block from downtown Evanston. A short walk to the elevated would take me downtown to my new auditor's position at Peat, Marwick, Mitchell.

That first Autumn I had a breakthrough experience while attending Northwestern's 1958 homecoming parade. Their homecoming weekend was my first Rah-Rah very classic campus experience, and it felt wonderful. Finally I was a part of a true university culture, and was experiencing something that had been missing during my commuting college years. I was still naïve, guarded and certainly not aggressive enough to jump in and to make new friends, but that would change.

Sitting one night in my friend Bob's car, I became frustrated that our relationship still had not turned sexual. I got up enough nerve to say directly to Bob "let's go to bed." I had to do this to make this happen because he was a rather conservative guy with southern social graces and he apparently was not one to instigate action. He flinched at my boldness, but nevertheless we broke the ice sexually as a result of my action. We became better friends, and later that year I suggested that we become roommates, which we did. My domestic life had begun. Bob gave me some fashion advice based on his old guard Southern upbringing. "Always buy the best quality clothing, it lasts a long time and is always in good taste." So I went down to Brooks Brothers and bought two wool suits that I would wear at my first job and for many years to come.

Bob's guidance also helped me find the social centers of activity so I could meet people my first months in Evanston. Those connections helped fire up my new gay lifestyle with gusto. The main areas to meet other gay men were "The Bushes," a cruise park south of campus on the lakefront, the basement bathroom at Deering library on campus, and "The Hut" coffee house just south of campus. The Hut was a somewhat notorious hangout that attracted many students from the Music school, Theater and English departments. I took full advantage of all of those venues throughout the year.

Bob and I met often at The Hut, which became my social hangout. It was a favorite of semi-bohemians connected with the university and I found the people there exotic and interesting. A lot of students hung out at The Hut and it occurred to me that some of them were probably gay. Bob would make comments about certain individuals from time to time so that I was able to hone my "gaydar."

One night I saw a cute guy in a white tee shirt leave The Hut. Eventually we met and I developed a crush on Bruce during the summer of 1958. One evening I was alerted in my attic room by some small pellets hitting the window. Bruce was down below my third story room in order to get my attention-- and my attention he did get.

Through Bruce and Bob I met many other local men who broadened me tremendously on the lifestyles of the mostly upper middle class guys that were abundant in the town. I was learning fast after each new introduction, and the introductions often developed into sexual liaisons. Gradually through word of mouth it became known that I was a new face around campus.

In Evanston, the chic thing was to live in a coach house. There were lots of them in Evanston on the grounds of huge homes built early in the century. Wally, a teacher at Evanston High School, lived in a coach house in South Evanston, and it became a delightful place to meet more friends. Evanston

High School and some of its staff were a major force in the gay milieu in town. Theater, musicals, costuming, and actors were discussed freely in his coach house setting.

Another group that Bruce introduced me to was in an impressive coach house just off campus. Ken was the set designer for Northwestern University's theatrical productions, and therefore the college group that gathered around him was cultured, and so cool. One afternoon he played for us a 33-rpm recording of a recently opened Broadway musical. It had brilliant music and lyrics that told a story. The musical was *Candide*, based on Voltaire's story of attained and then unattained happiness, and it had music by Leonard Bernstein. Well, I was hooked. This crowd was obviously plugged into the Broadway circuit, NYC and all that jazz. Soon afterwards I was invited by Ken to come back for an afternoon of wild sensual abandon at his townhouse. I had arrived.

Evanston was the site of an intense and rewarding interaction between students, residents and university teachers and staff during the sixties. That scene made a tremendous impression on me. I was meeting a whole new world of people. This is what had been missing in my life in my years up to then.

18. MEETING THE MAN

One evening in April 1959 I decided to take a walk after an evening at The Hut. The talk in town was that there was cruising in the evenings on the downtown streets, so I thought I would see if there was anybody around. I was convinced that I would need to be more aggressive if I was to meet more people. As I turned onto Sherman Avenue, I noticed someone across the street. A guy was standing in a dimly lit alcove in front of Kresge's dime store. Hmm. I wonder if he is gay. I approached him and made myself known. "How are you? I asked. "It's a nice night, isn't it?" We started a conversation and I suggested that we take a walk to enjoy the balmy night weather. I learned he was a student in the School of Music who was just finishing his junior year. His name was Denis. I suggested a date for the next afternoon and he told me to meet him at the music rehearsal building. I was excited to have made my first proper date. Denis was waiting in front of the building and we spent time together walking and talking, about ourselves and our interests. We set up another date to go to the Varsity Theater to see *Mein Uncle*, a foreign film of great boredom. During the film, we touched lightly and electric waves of excitement rushed through my body. I invited him to my apartment and we had our first sexual experience. Our relationship grew from there and we started seeing each other on a regular basis. Denis was a delightful person, sexy in his way, and he made me feel wanted.

I mentioned my new friend to my roommate Bob, and he apparently knew about Denis, and heard that he had broken up with a fellow student,

Steve, with whom he had shared an apartment for a time. I was a bit dismayed that he already had a previous relationship. Probably my Catholic upbringing about staying with your spouse forever and exclusively? Somehow this old-fashioned concept passed from my mind quickly as I pursued my relationship with Denis.

Denis was a local boy. He had returned to live with his parents at their home in Wilmette just a few miles up the road north of Evanston. Eventually, he mentioned that he was a pianist and performing with the orchestra at the upcoming *Waa-Mu Show*, the major musical variety show staged each year on campus. He told me that he had composed two songs that would accompany skits in the show. Lyrics were by Steve, when they had collaborated some months earlier. Did I want a ticket to the performance? You bet I did. The show was exciting, and in addition I was dually impressed that I was having a relationship with not only a compatible guy but a musical talent as well.

Denis and I became regulars and we saw each other often. I was thrilled to have someone that I could consider a full time and permanent friend and lover, who could be a foundation for my life. It seemed a healthy and satisfying way to live my life.

We went on several outings and dates, including one memorable afternoon for a beach picnic on the sand by the shores of Lake Michigan. It was on a small strip of sandy beach at the southernmost tip of campus. We ate our sandwiches and took pictures. Denis surprised me soon afterward with a small picture album with some very loving thoughts about me and our budding relationship.

This was a turning point and foreshadowed a new seriousness for us. I would often pick him up at school and take him to his Wilmette home. It was a thrilling courtship.

Denis would visit me in my attic apartment that I shared with my roommate Bob. One most memorable time I was laid up with a cold and for my birthday Denis surprised me by bringing his new recording of the Broadway musical *Gypsy* starring the icon Ethyl Merman as Mama Rose. We sat transfixed as the story unfolded through the music and lyrics. Julie Stein had written a beautiful score and to this day that cast recording represents the most intriguing story telling musical album of all time. I want the music played at my funeral. I would often dance around my apartment and kick high to that music, and eventually to other thrilling Broadway music of the time.

One evening, in my Studebaker, Denis and I had a serious conversation about our developing feelings. I think it was I that suggested a long term permanent lover relationship. It seemed like the time was right to commit to one another. As we talked, I held back a bit, knowing realistically that I could not promise to be totally faithful sexually. On that basis, Denis and I agreed to make our bond permanent. We became "lovers," the term of the times. It was the summer of 1959.

After that we needed to do some fine tuning as it related to sex with other people. Both of us had been sexually active up to that time with men we had met in the usual places. I continued to cruise the park. He did the same. In fact shortly thereafter, we met at the park the first time after our bond commitment, and it was a bit awkward, but over time as we agreed, our extracurricular activities became a natural part of our lives, and when either of us met someone particularly nice we would often invite them back again to see both of us. As a result, our social group expanded rapidly.

There was a funny situation very early on when I discovered that Denis did not know how to drive nor did he have a driver's license. Amazing at twenty-two! So I took him out in my stick shift Studebaker and tutored him on how to drive. The tricky part of shifting gears was coordinating the clutch pedal with the gear changes, and how to finesse this with concurrent use of the accelerator pedal. We were using a major street, Green Bay Road for the training. And Denis drove as I was giving intelligent advice. As he approached a stop sign on a very slight incline, he killed the engine. The car stopped and it started slowly drifting backward. Panic! Soon he got hand and foot coordinated and we were able to safely cross the intersection. I was a bit angry that he screwed up.

During the course of his last year at Northwestern Denis continued living at home and I occasionally visited and met his family. We often had holiday meals at their home. We even managed a few sexual liaisons in his bedroom suite upstairs.

After Denis graduated he moved out from his Wilmette home and we were able to live together for the first time. The summer of 1960 we decided to look for our own apartment. We mentioned to our friend Jack, our intention to move and he said that he owned a two flat that had an attic apartment that we could afford. Denis and I moved in, with a rent of $135 a month. We now had our very own place.

We soon invited my ex roommate Bob, and his two friends, Kenny and

"Puss" to our first entertaining at our new apartment. I am sure they were underwhelmed by the modesty of our abode, because they were used to somewhat more elegant surroundings. Bob's friends were real characters and their opinions were eye openers for me, as I am sure mine were to them. The boys were all very helpful in acquainting me with the joys of the old South. They piqued our interest enough for us to plot our first motor excursion into the southland.

During this time when Denis finished college, and began his first teaching job, I was working at accounting jobs that I hated. By 1961 I found a better job downtown at Brunswick Corporation in the International Division. This was a job where I was still very reluctant to take any creative initiative. Once again, I was ill at ease in the corporate world but I stuck it out for two years. More than ever I wanted to work "closer to home."

19. EVANSTON – THE SOCIAL SCENE

The sixties were a once in a lifetime decade during which I discovered the joy of community with like-minded people. Life in Evanston was full of exuberance, and the gay lifestyle was in full swing, even though most gay guys were in the closet to the rest of the world. It was the perfect town and gown situation where working professionals, academics, students, and liberal thinkers could thrive. The educated and decidedly young, gay, community wanted to have a good time, and we succeeded. Denis and I started our life-long relationship in this milieu. We were committed to one another, and we were open to all kinds of relationships with others without qualms.

One of our first invitations as a couple was from a well healed gay professional who had an impressive home in town. We were not yet members of the upscale in-crowd but we were invited because Denis was known to be an excellent pianist, and I was invited as his partner. The host specified musical entertainment, so Denis and some fellow students were engaged to be the entertainment. Their musical gig was a big success and we all enjoyed the camaraderie, and had a great time. I envied the host's baby blue high pile, wall-to-wall carpeting, that was most popular and trendy at the time.

Another man about town and a notorious party thrower was Jack. He had a great coach house on an alley just west of the "L" near downtown Evanston. Jack was three or four years older than we were and he knew lots of people. He was known by virtually everyone in the gay scene on the North Shore. Jack was the adopted son of a local judge and he was raised in an impressive Evanston home as a child. Jack was gay, but closeted from his parents, even though he lived a most active gay life around town. Evanston's largest and most raucous parties took place at his coach house on a regular basis. There was always a buzz in town about an upcoming party there. Jack knew a particularly eclectic group of people. Somehow the word got out to the Chicago gay crowd and to people from far and wide around the Chicago area. Some military guys were guests, mainly sailors from Great Lakes Naval Air station located north of Evanston. There were nellies and butches from all over, but no drag queens that I remember. A few women. Ages of the crowd ranged from eighteen to sixty. More than once I met someone that I hooked up with. At these parties, I often had one beer too many but always had a great time, and I met some intriguing people from all over the Chicago area.

I continued attending parties at Wally' coach house, now with Denis at my side. These parties were a bit more subdued than Jack's, but intriguing and educational nevertheless. Occasionally there might be a high school student or someone who had just graduated in attendance. Definitely eighteen years old, I think. Often in attendance was Frank, a mature older faculty member who was in charge of costuming for the high school's dramatic productions. Frank had a maturity and a wealth of knowledge, a strong artistic sense, and a flare for magnificence in costuming. He was a great story teller as well, and was the first person I knew who was an intelligent "camp." In addition, Frank provided a level of informed gossip that I had never been exposed to before.

There was expectant sensuality at Wally's place but rarely any overt sexual action. I do remember a particularly beautiful boy, who had graduated from Evanston High School, who had extensive involvement in their theatrical productions. His name was Steve. Steve had beautiful long straight hair and fine features. Party goers would get a bit tipsy, and, on one occasion and Steve and I wound up in the bedroom together on the floor. I was not aggressive enough to reach out to him and nothing occurred except a forbidden sort of unfulfilled relationship. Many years later after he had spent time in New York City, our paths would again cross in San Francisco, and under surprising circumstances, where he worked as a sex club attendant.

Mark was another high school graduate that I met at Wally's coach house. He was a voluptuous young man, who according to word of mouth, was fantastically hung. One time, I was chauffeuring Mark in my car, and was waiting for an invitation to have sex, but it never came, and I was too reluctant to make an independent aggressive move with him. Years later I heard that he moved to New York City and became one of many legendary dominant tops in the extreme sex circles of the big apple.

At one point, I received an invitation to go to a party in Hyde Park, home of the University of Chicago, on the South Side. A group of us drove down in one car and we were ushered into a huge Edwardian mansion which was the home of Hugh, a slightly older guy who had lots of very young friends, perhaps hustlers. Lots of sexual vibes there, and again I had several beers too many and missed out on some of the more wild action as the party developed. During the long drive home on Lake Shore Drive I was blotto, and only semi-aware that I had slumped to the floor by the back seat. After that experience I vowed to pace my drinking, so that I could have a buzz, but still be alert to what was happening. (I had to remind myself to heed Brother John's advice about "MODERATION.")

20. NEW HOME – FRESH OPPORTUNITIES

In 1961 I noticed a rental sign in my daily walk to the "L" station. A townhouse apartment was being renovated and the door was open so I walked in. The place was charming and it contained a stairway to the second-floor bedrooms. A stairway, my first! Rent was $185 a month, considerably more than what we were currently paying but I was so excited about the space I took Denis over immediately and we decided to stretch our budgets to afford it. It turned out that the rental agent did not want two early twenties something roommates in that unit but said we should look at the end unit which was also vacant. Apparently, the managing agent thought that as young men, if we were noisy we would be better off at the end of this six-unit building. In 1962 Denis and I moved in and set about to furnish it and make it our home. We lived there for the rest of the decade.

Although Denis and I had jobs, neither of us was secure about our financial situation. I started getting into debt immediately after graduation from Loyola. We were using our credit cards to buy basic first-time needs such as suits for work, and furniture, and car repairs.

About this time our previous landlord, Jack, tipped me off about a book that was a big best seller at the time called "How to turn $1,000 into One Million Dollars in Real Estate." That book whetted my interest and I began to believe that real estate investing was a way to break my reliance on jobs that did not fulfill me. I was impressed with another idea that one could use leverage and a low down payment to get started in real estate. I scoured the small ads in our local newspaper for opportunities to purchase with a low down payment and I noticed an ad that said "$500 down with the owner to carry a loan at favorable terms." We met with the owner who liked us and was impressed that we both had jobs, and were ambitious enough to pursue our dreams. The investment property was a brick two flat building just off campus on Ridge Avenue. We scraped up the $500 down payment with difficulty, paying some of it in monthly installments. This allowed us to complete the purchase. We now owned our first piece of real estate.

After the purchase of this building I got the real estate bug big time, and decided to study for my real estate license to become a real estate agent. I was not happy working for others and felt lost in the corporate world and thought I could increase my income doing something I actually liked.

Soon after obtaining my license, I set out to join the staff of an established, local real estate company. With lots of persistence I approached them repeatedly, generally making myself an annoyance until they agreed to accept me on their staff. Apparently, I did not fit their usual salesperson's profile because I was single and a new North Shore resident with no actual selling experience. Theirs was an old-line downtown business whose owners were Christian Scientists.

Once they approved me I went to work taking sales calls which I expected would be my main source of clients. I knew no one socially who had money or an interest in purchasing real estate. Gradually I was able to work with buyers and had my first successes. Through a friend, I was put in touch with a Mrs. Z. She was in her sixties and owned an Edwardian mansion that sat right on the lakefront in Evanston. With the help of my broker. I listed the property for sale, which subsequently provided my biggest commission to date. My relationship with Mrs. Z led to another referral.

By my second year with my Evanston broker I surprisingly had amassed enough commissions to earn $10,000 that year. I was the highest-earning agent in the company of twelve sales people and it was an apparently a shock to the rest of the experienced staff. I eventually found out that during my "Floor Time," when taking incoming inquiries that all calls were being monitored by the receptionist, and she was instructed to bypass the floor agent on any calls from a property owner wanting to list their property for sale. The one call that did slip through to me garnered me a nice commission. When I found this out I was unnerved and thought that I would have better support from working at another brokerage. It was time to try to move to a bigger more prestigious firm based on my successful earnings in 1963. I attracted the attention of a premier firm that had several offices along the North Shore. I also learned that they had our friend Jack on their staff as a part time agent! One of their agents was assigned to vet me over dinner. During that meeting, I dropped my guard and mentioned living with a roommate. The agent seemed sophisticated and pleasant, but no offer to join was forthcoming. I later surmised that they suspected I was gay and, for that conservative era, it was a too risky to have a gay person on their staff. My earnings took a precipitous dip later that year and I became desperate financially. I reluctantly decided that I needed to earn a salary as an accountant again.

21. TRAVELS WITH DENIS

Our very first road trip after moving into our townhouse was a foray to Atlanta for Easter. When we arrived in Atlanta we hit the gay bars instinctively, and immediately met a most festive group of gay natives. We attended a round of parties, where huge hats, semi-drag and dancing on pianos were the order of the day.

On to Miami where we checked into a modest motel in Miami Beach. We met lots of natives who introduced us to the gay scene in town. There was a sprinkling of gay bars in Miami Beach, usually located in neighborhoods that were more than a bit frayed. I met a gorgeous blond boy who took me to a lush square in Coconut Grove in mainland Miami, and he invited me to ride rear saddle on his motor bike. We scooted around town with utter abandon. That ride was terribly exhilarating, a bit scary but emotionally rewarding because I was tooting around with a beautiful boy. No Complaints.

Some of our travels involved situations closer to home. Milwaukee and Madison had gay scenes and were an easy drive for a weekend away. The Antlers Hotel in Milwaukee was notorious as a place where unbridled sex took place. Denis and I decided on separate rooms. I would walk the halls a lot. Denis often stayed in his room with an open door while making lesson plans and at the same time checking out the action.

Madison, Wisconsin, home of the University of Wisconsin, was another active community infused with a great mix of students, faculty and other likeminded people. Madison had a free spirit but the scene was decidedly mixed, with the gay crowd subtly fitting in. While cruising a campus john I met a student, Bob S. who filled us in on the gay scene there. Our paths would intertwine in Chicago and San Francisco in the coming years.

On our Wisconsin trips, we would often visit my grandma at her Lake Delavan cottage. She loved seeing us. We stayed in the attic and we had quiet sex several times. Quite a change from my childhood experiences there.

22. BOUNCY VISITS TO THE EAST COAST

We decided we had to get to the Big Apple and while in NYC we made sure we saw *Gypsy* with Ethyl Merman. That recording had been so iconic in our first year together. We also had tickets to see Barbra Streisand in *Funny Girl*, she being a new comer to the musical scene. We were wowed by both of those stars in those Broadway classic roles.

New York was madness times two. So many people on the streets. So much energy. We met with my flirtatious friend Bruce, who I had met that first Evanston summer. He moved to New York City after graduation and took a job as editor for a New York-based magazine. He graciously invited us to join him and his friends in New York that summer on Fire Island. We had heard about that resort and were excited to see what sex and sin the scene offered, that we could not experience back in the Midwest. Was it really better there? The plan was to travel to Fire Island and we would sleep over in a cottage that had been rented by a group of with-it Manhattan "A" gays. We travelled with our luggage by train to the Fire Island station and took a ferry to Cherry Grove, which was the trendiest and most popular gay community on the island in the mid-sixties and which we assumed was where we would be going. However, we discovered that our destination was the Pines, one community over. At the time the Pines was the more discrete gay community, yet an easy hike to the loud dance and sex scene in Cherry Grove. When we arrived, we were welcomed by a scintillating group of hot Manhattan men. We slept on the floor. We flirted. We did our walks over to the action in the Grove. The conversation was urbane, East Coast and cosmopolitan. These guys were classy; they worked in the Big Apple, and had glamourous jobs. In fact, the guys were so classy that they were generally unapproachable.

There was another East Coast gay resort that we visited twice. We had heard about from our Chicago friends, and they said it was a rival to Fire Island. Provincetown, Massachusetts. Our flight from Boston was in a cool, small plane to the Cape. We absolutely loved the safety, and secure feeling of gay isolation that this historic place embodied. Provincetown was in its heyday and was as charming and friendly a place as could be imagined. It had small town ambiance along with lots of early American history. It was absolutely swarming with relaxed gay guys having a ball. We stayed upstairs at an inn which showcased a bar and performance venue on the ground floor. The sounds of the shows wafted into our room. All in all, there was total magic to our time on the cape. What a joy being there.

One day a group of us travelled to a local pond that was popular with the gay set. When we arrived, I was overwhelmed by the beauty and serenity of the place. It had the look and the feel of Walden Pond. The experience was like being enveloped inside of a fairy tale. We left Provincetown with an enhanced feeling that there was a ground swell happening in the country, that gay life was coming out of the closet, and that we were an integral part of a national acceptance of our community, each place with its own special twist.

23. PARTIES, PARTIES

By the early'60s we were well known in the Evanston gay community. We had met lots of guys so we decided to throw our first party. We decided on a French theme, so we created decorations with Tri Colors and covered our gold silk draperies with them. The gathering was wildly successful. Our guest list included many students, and other young men from the area. Many were students in the Arts. Usually the guests were encouraged to BYOB (Bring Your Own Bottle) to keep costs down. Our musically talented friends were encouraged to sing and perform.

Our next party had a Broadway theme, and we featured a staircase scene for our friend Phil, so that he could make his grand entrance down our stairway. I will never forget his flamboyant entrance, holding an umbrella, and sashaying down our staircase, as he teased us with the rousing tune "Stairway to Paradise." As the sixties moved on we followed up with more parties with elaborate themes. Most of these morphed into impromptu after-party sexual scenes (Orgies) for people who stayed late. The upstairs bed and the downstairs living room rug were put to convenient use. One time I invited a new friend to join me for more privacy, and we pulled down the utility stairway to our attic storage. I threw a tee shirt haphazardly over the bare light bulb for more romantic lighting, and as he and I started our encounter we smelled smoke. We looked up and the tee shirt was on fire, so we scurried to put it out, fanned out the smoke, and triumphantly returned to the crowd.

Another memorable time, Jack Stillman, later to be porn star Jack Wrangler, a cute, blond twink student at the time, was semi naked near me on our olive green living room rug. I heard later that he felt self-conscious about his legs being too thin, so he always kept his pants on. I approached to touch him but was rejected. Too bad. Jack was a Theater school undergraduate and we struck up a somewhat aloof friendship. Denis and I lost touch with Jack after we moved from Evanston. Sometime later we were amazed that he had gone into gay porn films under the name of Jack Wrangler. He was very well known in those early years as a trail blazer in that business. Jack was somewhat of a mystery in Evanston, not fully out but gay for sure. He claimed then that he was the son of Dolores Grey, a musical actress who had done some Hollywood films. We learned later that this was y not true. Later we did find out that his father was a Hollywood producer, so there was a bit of truth for his claiming a Hollywood connection. Years later we chanced upon him in San Francisco at PS, a glitzy, mirrored Polk Street restaurant. He was with an older companion and Jack seemed genuinely surprised and impressed that Denis and I were successful and looked marvelously happy.

Denis kept a detailed record of our parties and of all our guests during those years; what we served, who RSVP'd and what beverages we had. I asked Denis to provide me with a list of attendees at our parties during the 1960s and a total of 274 men were documented as having been at our celebrations! Some of these men found their way into our beds or became conquests in various places around the city. Yes, we were very busy!

Liquor and beer were our drinks of choice. No cannabis or any hard drugs were being used to our knowledge. "Poppers," amyl nitrite, was the sexual enhancer of choice. Poppers were pharmaceutically correct in those days being a capsule that you snapped and sniffed. Many of us had had silver bullets (made of tin) into which the cracked open ampules were inserted to keep the ingredients fresh and easy. We often wore the chained bullets around our necks. Oh the simple depravity of it all. More serious goodies came later in the 1970s.

24. PROFESSIONAL LIFE – PREPARATIONS TO LEAVE CHICAGO

As an auditor with Bell and Howell in 1964 and 1965, I traveled to the West Coast and my eyes were opened to the attractions of California's gay scene. I explored both San Francisco and Los Angeles. Both cities appeared to be considerably more open, advanced and savvy than the Midwest. Although I was quite happy living in Evanston, the California lifestyle had that extra something that excited me. It was daring and even more outrageous than the scene in the Midwest. Denis and I made several vacation trips to California during the mid-60s, and he too liked what he saw. In addition to its West Coast locations my employer had a warehouse in upstate New York. When travelling on business the perks allowed me to enjoy the gay life as well in New York City.

Because I wanted a job closer to home that did not involve travelling, I interviewed for a position at Northwestern University in the Auditing department and was hired. The pace at the university was more laid back and I could go home for lunch and even walk to work if I wanted to.

In 1967 shortly after joining Northwestern, Chicago had an epic snow storm. The entire city was shut down and I took advantage of the day off to shoot pictures while taking a day-long walk around Evanston and the lake shore parks and campus. The scene was unbelievably beautiful with the white snow covering a hushed landscape. The snow was so high that I had to take each step independently and deliberately, and apparently unnaturally. Within 24 hours I was feeling discomfort in my hips and legs. Soon I could not walk and wound up on crutches for several weeks, and for a time I hobbled up and down the stairs to my Northwestern job.

One of the last icy Chicago challenges, we experienced in the winter of 1968. We had tickets to the opera and to save money on parking we decided to look for a place to park on the street just west of the river across from the Opera House. We braved the walk over the Washington Street Bridge and with the wind and the freezing temperature we practically froze in the three blocks to the theater. We knew after that incident that we wanted a life in a more comfortable climate.

Denis and I started talking and planning to leave the horrible cold winters and move to the West Coast. We put our investment duplex on the market and sold it for a profit of $6,000 on an initial investment of $500. That cash was a nest egg that we salted away as down payment for our next home. We now were prepared to make our move.

Honestly though, the main impetus for us to move was the continued nightmarish cold weather in Chicago.

Denis and I travelled to San Francisco and Los Angeles in 1968 to sample the cities once again. On the flight home from the West Coast we discussed their relative appeal. We loved them both. At the time, there was some bad press about the LA police department and they were known to raid the bars regularly, and generally make life difficult for the gay crowd. This concern was the tie breaker. On the plane we decided to move to San Francisco.

In Evanston, there was a seminal scene that took place one year before our departure. It is etched in my memory. One cold January night in 1969 I met a fellow who invited me to his nearby apartment. He asked me if I would like to smoke some marijuana. Yes, I did. He was surprised that at 32, I had never had it. So he became my mentor and I became his student. His challenge was to make my first smoke and the night a memorable one. He rolled a joint and he gave it to me at which point I told him that I did not know how to inhale. My host assured me and guided me as I sucked in air from the joint and practiced my first inhale. He then inhaled. I took another hit. He took another hit. I took a third hit and I said that I did not feel anything different. Then a pause and my very first sweet cannabis rush started to make my head buzz. This brought back the memory of my fist alcohol rush at the age sixteen, while drinking Mogen David wine on Christmas Eve after midnight mass. A few more tokes of MJ and a sweet, mellow, serene high followed. All this made the sexual experience of the evening superb. Afterwards my host proceeded to set out a tray of fruit and cheese, as he explained that I would have the munchies. I did not, because I was just too happy experiencing the high.

I made one last trip to San Francisco in April of 1970 to scout out potential living arrangements and found a place for us to live. I had scouted the neighborhoods and saw a for-sale sign on a building on the fringe of the Haight Ashbury and above the Eureka Valley, soon to be called "The Castro." I excitedly called Denis from an outdoor phone booth to tell him what I had found. Denis said "let's buy the building." He flew out and we cemented our purchase.

We used our nest egg of $6,000 to make the down payment and we signed a contract of sale which gave us time to qualify for a new loan after we became established and were employed. We now were ready to take up residence in San Francisco and were about to change completely the direction of our lives. I had a goal to continue my quest to be successful in a field that I believed in, and this quest would propel me into the business world of Real Estate.

Hello to San Francisco

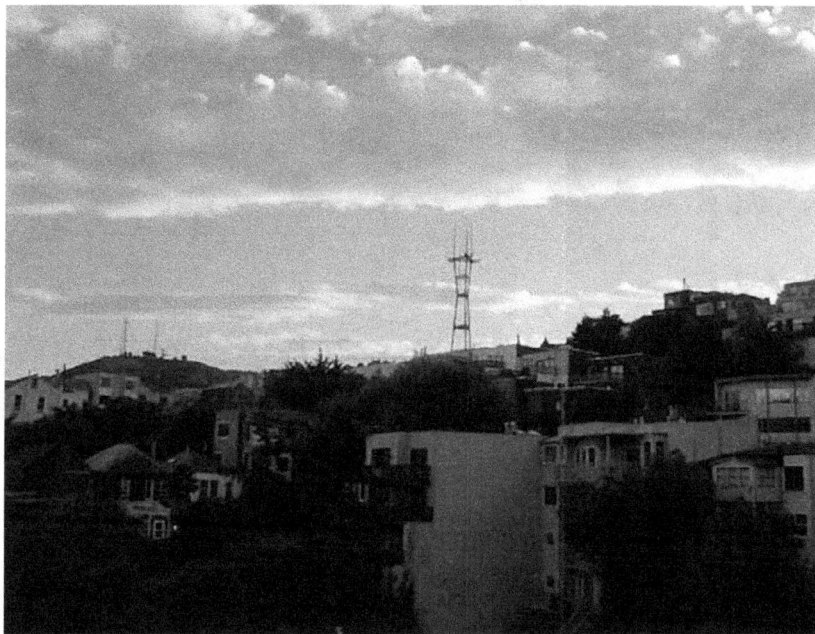

Twin Peaks Sutro Tower, San Francisco.

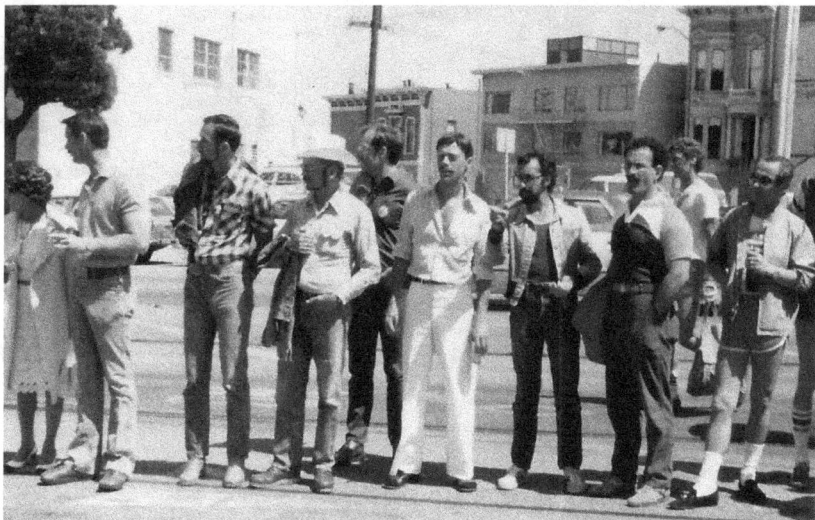

Mid-Market, watching and waiting for the Tricycle Race. I'm in white!

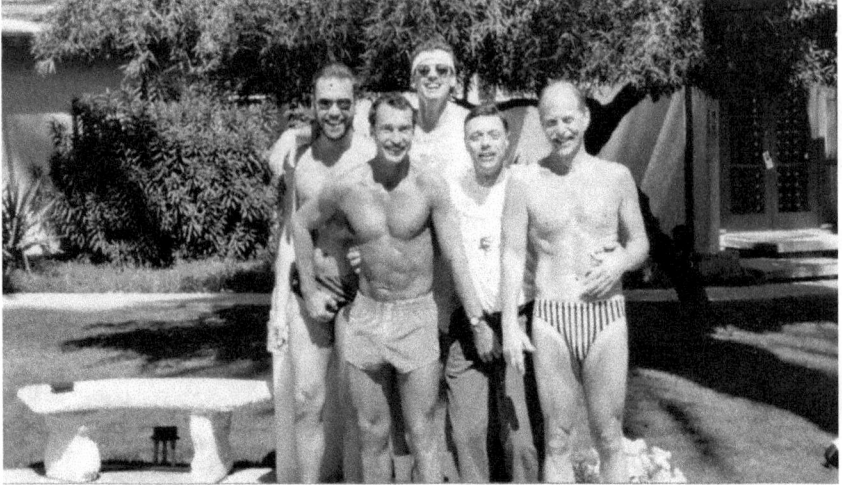

First getaway in Palm Springs at Dave's Villa Caprice, 1970s. (How short I am!)

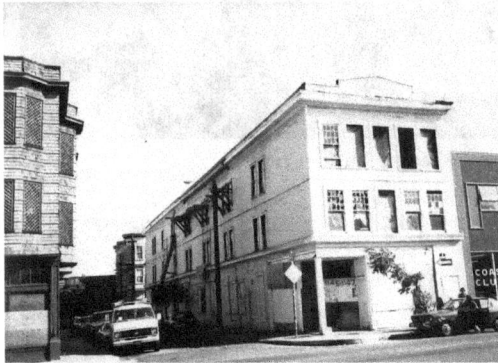

SOMA South of Market sin spots.
The notorious Barracks and Red Star Saloon.

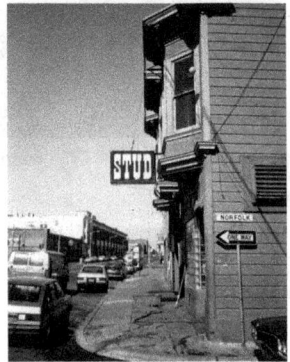

SOMA. Original Stud Bar,
1970s. A dream place.

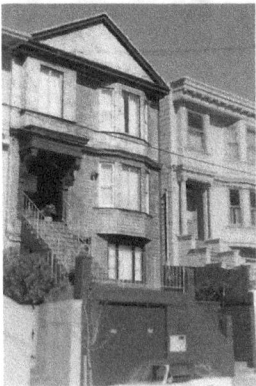

Our first San Francisco home,
on Buena Vista Hill.

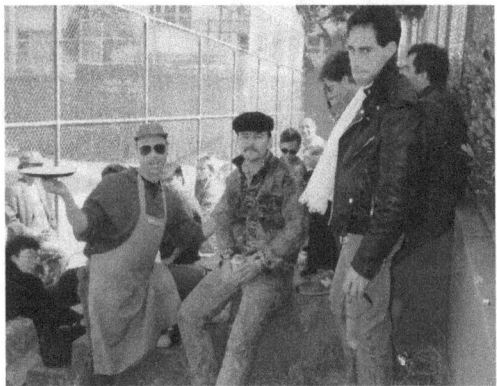

Moi, camping it up at Collingwood Park
softball event, 1980s.

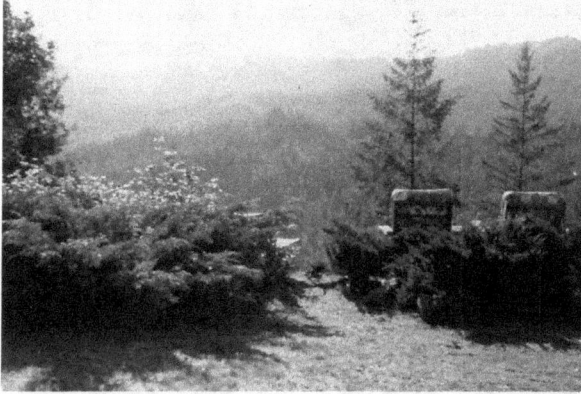

Julie Andrews Point, Wildwood Ranch, Russian River.

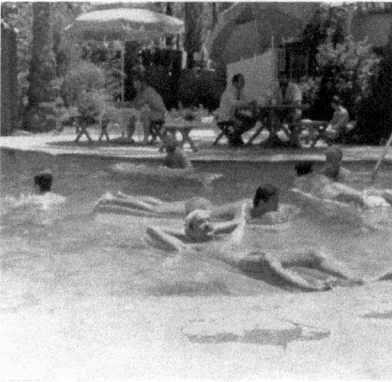

Typical laid back fun at pool, Russian River.

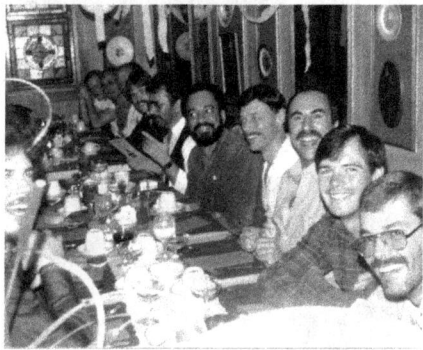

The Fabulous Fickle Fox staff dinner, 1978. Restaurant/cabaret showcasing Denis's piano talent.

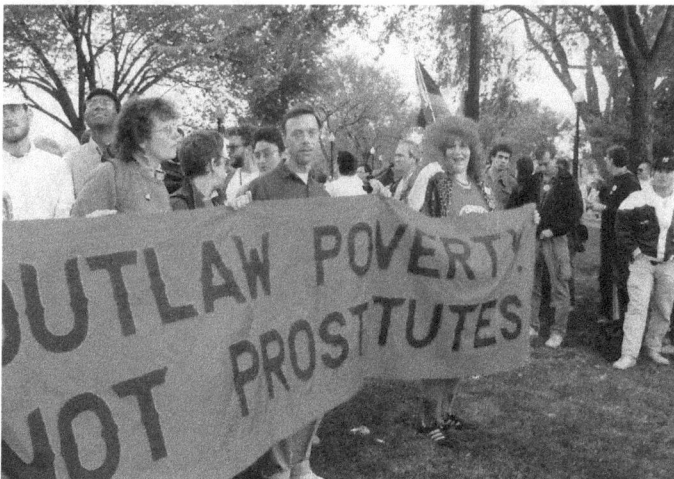

I finally got to march in the Gay Pride Parade, 1987 (note the banner).

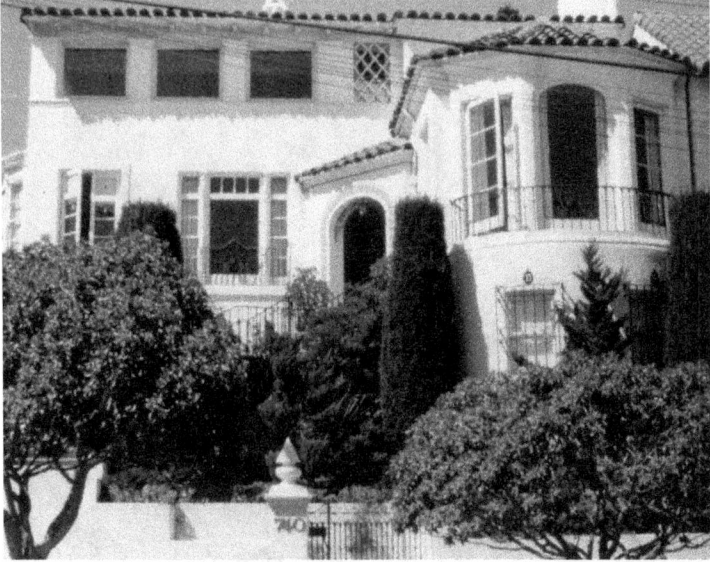

Our gem of a home overlooking Dolores Park, 1976.

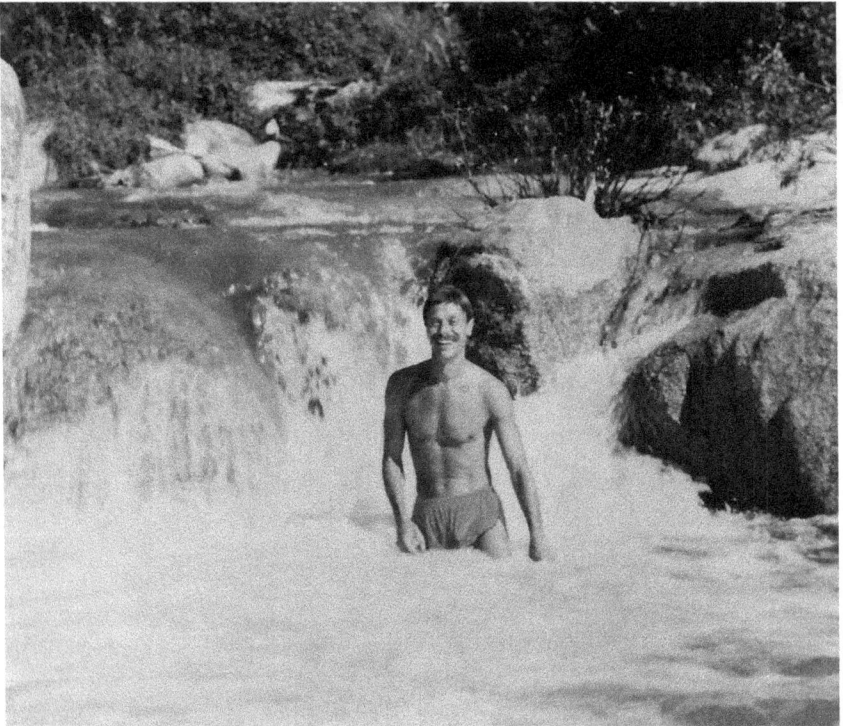

Puerto Vallarta, 1979. Spur of the moment trip with Joe.
My most glamorous scene, ever.

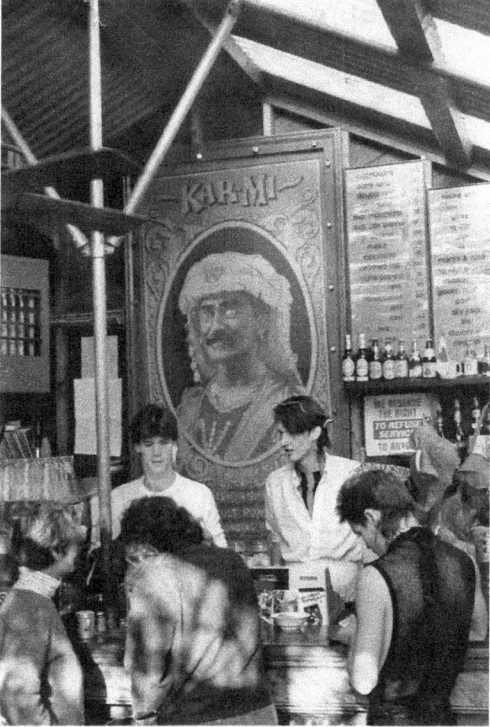

Café Flore, 1985. My new social world.

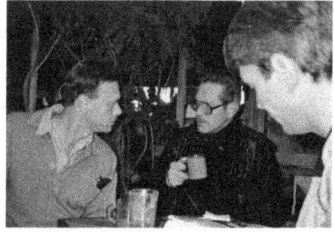

Intense conversation at the Café.

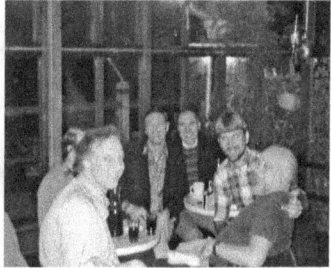

The gang at Café Flore.

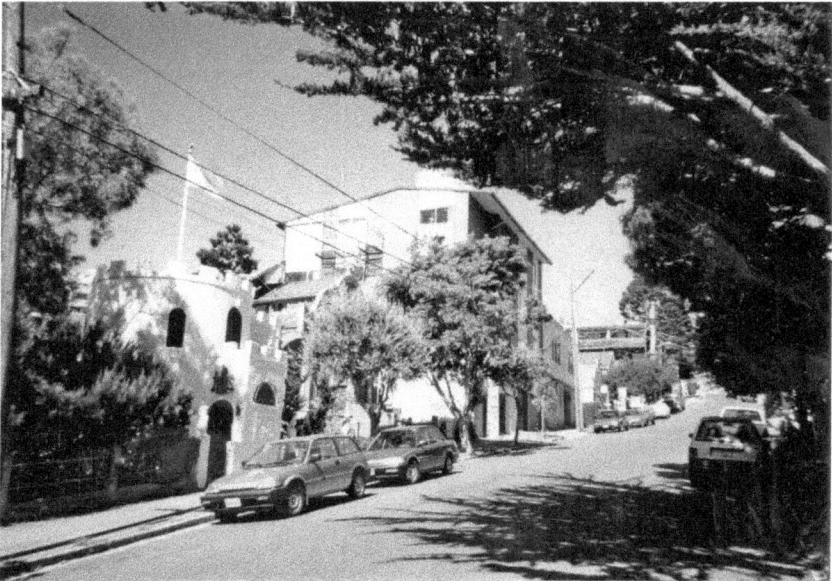

Our States Street Home for seventeen years.

Hello to Palm Springs

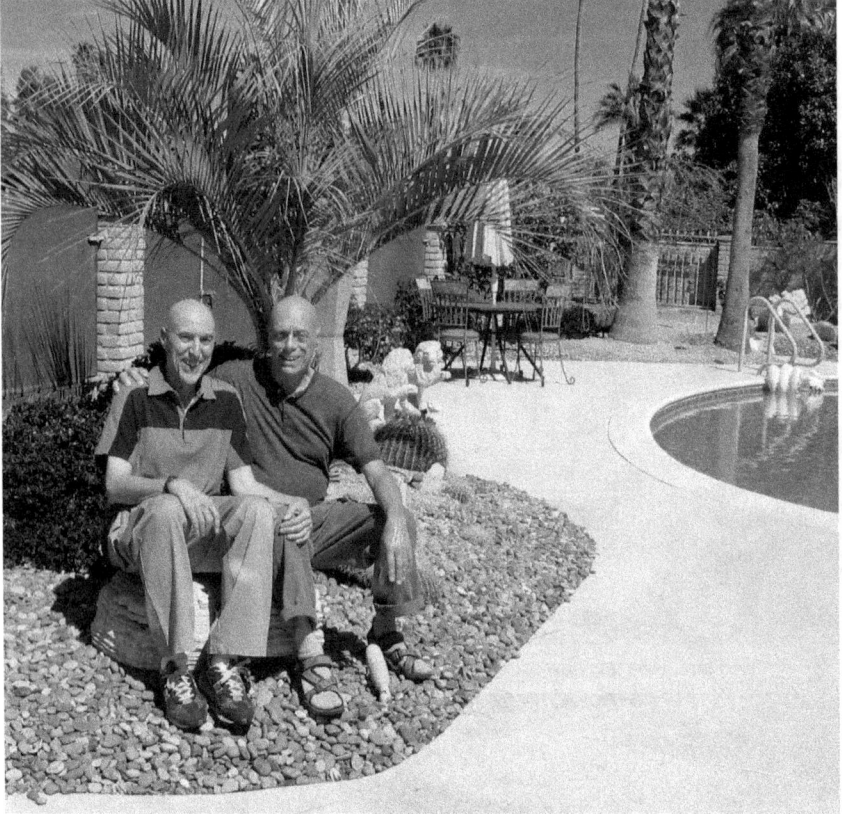

Fiftieth anniversary, 2009. In our Palm Springs garden.

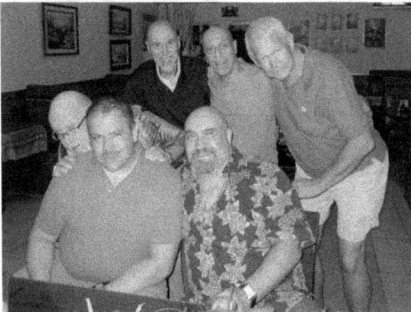

Koffi Café. "The Krazies."

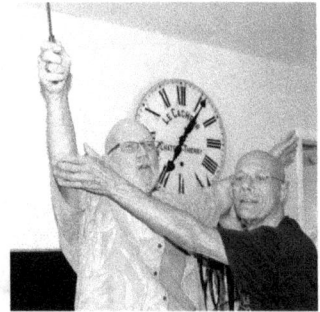

Herr Richard Hilgenberg directing.

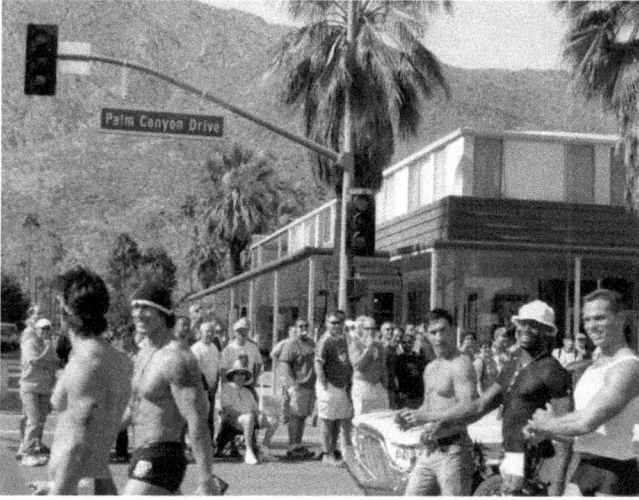

Cuties at Palm Springs gay parade.

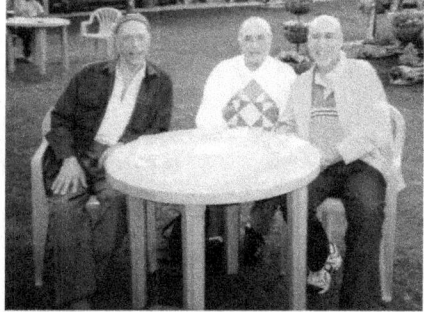

Rob, Empress Jose Sarria, Denis at Koffi.

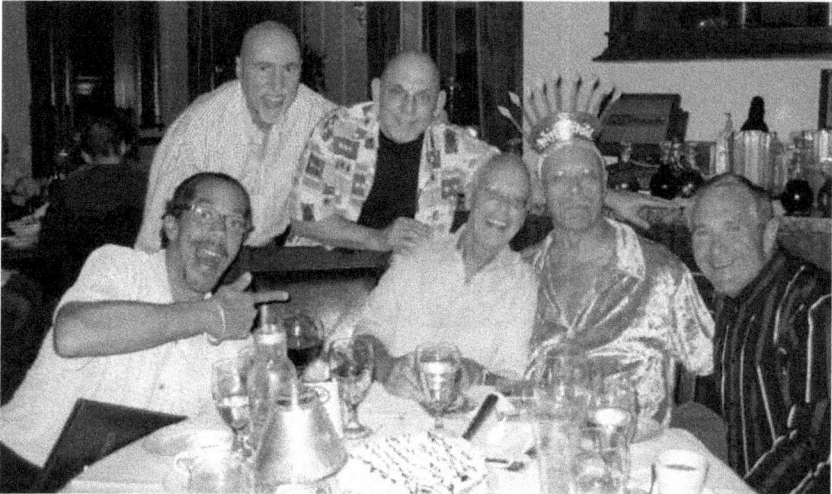

Rob's seventieth birthday, 2007.

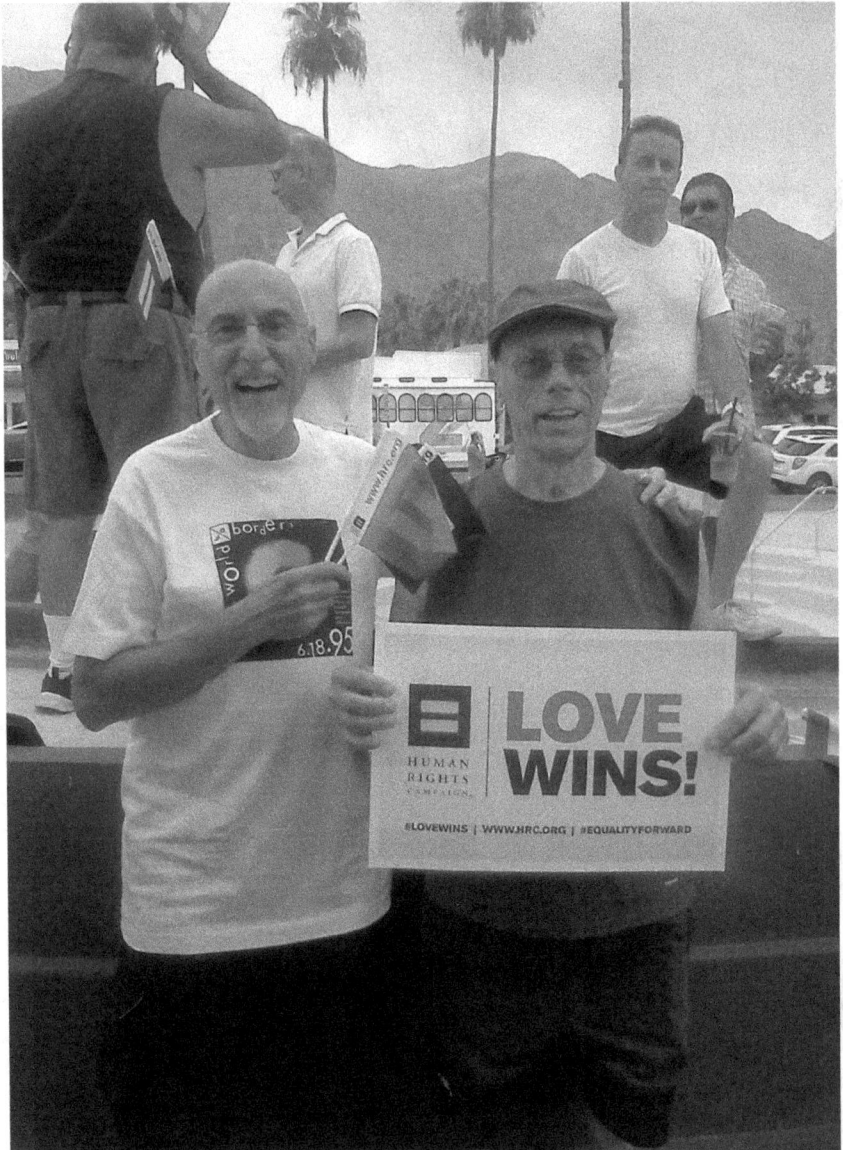

2015 Gay marriage installed in the USA.

25. INTRODUCTION TO THE 1970s

On the morning of June 17th, 1970, we approached San Francisco. That first sighting of the emerald city as we drove over the Oakland bay bridge was hypnotic. We had reached our OZ. We were now the proud owners of a three-flat building on Alpine Terrace, near Buena Vista Park. Ours was the top flat which had a rooftop view of the downtown and the East bay.

Believe it or not a milkman made deliveries to our front door. Three flights down, he set the milk bottles in a space hidden below the front outside stairway which we accessed through a small, discrete wooden door. Milk, butter, eggs were delivered to us there weekly. This service was right out of early Americana, a relic from the nineteenth century, and unbelievably these deliveries lasted into the early '70s.

Our property was on the east side of Buena Vista hill, a borderline neighborhood at that time, but buffered and caressed by Buena Vista Park. Our home was around the corner from the Haight Ashbury district but it seemed safely removed from that hectic, almost war-torn neighborhood. We had rooftop views and a one car garage that had been carved into the hillside soon after the historic 1906 earthquake when the structure was built. Alpine Terrace was a gem of a street, extremely quiet because it was only two blocks long and there was no through traffic.

Another advantage of our location was that Castro Street was nearby, where there was gay activity day and night. Several of our neighbors on Alpine Terrace were gay so our street was a welcoming place to live. The neighbor across the street, who we could see primping in front of his mirror, became known as "the hair lady." It looked like a man in front of the mirror, but emerging on the street, it was a person in women's clothing. The mystery was solved – or was it?

The bars on Castro Street down the hill were our neighborhood bars. Our favorite was the Pendulum on 18th Street. "The Pendulum Swings" was their motto. It was a block-buster of a place and it excited me the moment I first stepped in. The place boasted a much hopped up crowd, mostly beer drinkers, pretty masculine, but they also were loose enough to bounce to the music, and the guys were ready for sex. It was very informal and everyone was reveled in their sensuality.

One character who hung out at the front of the bar and who seemed to rule as if he was the owner, but he wasn't, was Peter King. Peter was in his late fifties, an old-school Chinese guy, gay, who had lived in the neighborhood for years. Very bubbly, easy to talk to, and worldly wise. He camped with everyone who came in including me. He owned a somewhat run-down cottage perched high in Dolores Heights, and he extended an invitation to me to discuss real estate valuation. Peter at the time was cash strapped and needed to refinance. As a thank you for my advice he gifted me a pair of ornate green onyx one-foot high objects. Not my taste but probably valuable heirlooms from his Chinese family. Many years later he wanted them back but I kept them!

26. A FREE AND EASY SUMMER

The summer of 1970 was the first time in my life that I did not have a job lined up. I started to interview for an accounting position at several hospitals, and I had a good introduction letter from my previous boss. This connection got me an interview for a controller's position at St. Joseph's hospital just two blocks up the hill. The interview went nowhere, probably because I was a lightweight and too young to take on that degree of responsibility. Curiously, St. Josephs closed several years later. I continued to apply to several other hospitals in the city hoping to get a job in the nonprofit sector.

Denis was also out of a job and our resources were dwindling, so Denis signed up to study for an advanced degree that would take him down to Stanford University. He felt he needed to have a Doctorate degree in Music in order to qualify for a California teaching job at a good school. He commuted by car and in the meantime he kept his eyes open for some paying work where he could use his valuable piano skills.

That first summer in San Francisco after we got settled into our flat, I found myself at liberty, as an adult, to enjoy my first summer where I was totally free all day and all week with no job to go to. I had time to meander afternoons around the neighborhood.

Nearby Buena Vista Park was known as an outdoor trysting and meeting place and I would drive up the winding road to a park at the top. Gay men were everywhere; in the parking lot, on the trails and in the bushes. All were looking for sex in the moment. This was a most popular daytime attraction in the neighborhood, where you could roam the hillside, meander through the bushes and get the feeling you were in a nature preserve, all in the heart of the city.

Down on Castro Street the sidewalks were becoming a fantasy promenade for young men. Where they came from I did not know. I began to meet some very laid back and free spirited men. Daytime walks became surreal. The business district was jumping with affable testosterone-charged and available men. At times, I could not believe it was real. It seemed more like a dream and too good to be true.

There was an eclectic array of gay bars in the Castro where one could step into different worlds just by stepping from the sidewalk through their doors that revealed a hothouse of men. Inside it was a circus, a celebration of youth.

The Midnight Sun was one of the first of the new bars to locate on Castro Street. It occupied the old space of the Bank of Italy which had moved out years earlier to their new Bank of America location down the block on Market Street. The façade of the old location was colonnaded with two iron columns at the entrance. Shortly after we arrived in the city, the Midnight Sun's interior was completely redecorated with a fantasy theme. There was an extremely narrow street frontage that widened once you entered. I could sit at the long bar with tight standing room only--- cheek to jowl intimate.

Toad Hall was another trailblazing bar. It was an eclectic place situated inside an old Victorian building near the corner of Castro and Eighteenth. The building held Star Pharmacy, which is Walgreens drug store today. Presiding over Star Pharmacy was an infamous clerk, Jackie Starr, who greeted every one coming in. She had the looks of a tall drag queen compete with bouffant hair style – but she was a woman, and straight.

The first time I walked into Toad Hall I could not believe the décor. The whole place, up to the high ceilings, was filled with three dimensional constructions that depicted an old children's tale. Every six months the entire bar theme was changed to something different, equally enthralling.

Twin Peaks Tavern. Suddenly this old Irish bar with the blocked-out windows was opened up with views to and from the streets. It was a bold move by the new owners. I would go there for a slightly more sedate experience. Once inside the openness seemed natural. The crowd was a bit more well-behaved because of the windows, but the electricity was palpable. There was a tiny mezzanine in the rear where you could hang out below it, or above the crowd. Eventually the place drew a large clientele of men who worked downtown, who came to imbibe and socialize after work.

On the weekends, I would go to a quirky gay owned place at the corner of Hartford and eighteenth streets called the Corner Grocery Store. There was a deli counter, and old wooden tables were randomly scattered throughout the room. Originally it was a butcher shop, and it still had meat hooks hanging from the ceiling. I enjoyed the classical music and the mini-stage live performances by local classical artists and singers.

These places were the beginning of the new Castro. Other gay owned and oriented businesses soon opened. I dropped in occasionally to the Jaguar bookstore during the day that had a back room for intimate encounters.

Other popular places were The Neon Chicken a restaurant on Eighteenth Street; The Obelisk that sold upscale objects. Flowers Etc. next to the Midnight Sun was owned by my friend Richard, who reminded me of this after I met him many years later in Palm Springs.

A long-time business that prospered in sync with the gay infusion was Cliff's Variety Store. It was a mainstay of the older residents but the enlightened owners changed their focus to glide with the times and embraced those changes.

The gay owned Gilded Age stocked an amazing array of English antiques and furniture, sent by the owner's mother back in England. It was a great place to browse and find authentic English pieces. I still have many to this day.

The young men attracted to the Castro were savvy and extremely horny. I was thirty-three, but many of the men coming into the Castro were ten years younger and often just out of college. They too were looking for a welcoming place to live their lives free from the constraints and boredom of their home towns.

In the evenings at the Pendulum bar, I began to meet some intriguing characters who were definitely more diverse than the men were in Chicago. This was California in the aftermath of the Summer of Love in the Haight Ashbury. Bell bottom pants, tie dies and long hair were still in abundance in the Castro. On the heels of the 1969 stonewall riots in New York, The San Francisco gay scene was taking off, and it built upon that seminal New York event. It promised gay men a new life of greater sexual freedom.

One of the most unusual men that I met at the Pendulum bar was Kenneth Marlowe. He was a forty-something handsome guy, who wore a wide brimmed leather hat as his signature. He, like Peter King, was a sophisticated veteran of many years in the active gay communities around the country. It turns out he had an alter ego as "Mister Madam," who was writing a book outlining his life as a transgender person. He was known in the neighborhood as a special person, with a history and persona to match. One night Kenneth and a group of us stayed until the bar closed and we walked around the corner to get some coffee and donuts. We were being a bit loud and flamboyant. A tipsy Irishman was coming out from one of the straight bars holding a bottle of beer, and out of nowhere he hit me in the face with his bottle. (The straight bars in the Castro were mostly "Irish bars.") Our group chased him away and they administered to my face, which luckily had only minor bruises. I was in shock, and unnerved, and feeling I had been discriminated against in my own new neighborhood. This encounter was the only violent altercation that I experienced during my time living in San Francisco. It soon became apparent to me that this kind of incident was the last gasp of the old guard, the straight Irish and German, long-time residents of the neighborhood. I realized then that they understandably resented the gay influx, and the massive changes that were occurring in their beloved Eureka Valley.

Sunday afternoons, Mr. Madam held informal showings of 8-millimeter porn films. I was invited by my Pendulum friends to join in. It was a convenient excuse to hitch up with someone in the mood for pleasure. I met Tom, a cute, short sandy-haired guy, and when I mentioned that I was unemployed he heartily recommended that I start to charge for sex to tide me over. He said it was fun and easy. Hmm, what an offer! Before long I was advertising in the *Berkeley Barb* and in the *Bay Area Reporter*, both of which had a large number of "model" ads in their classified sections.

Our rear apartment would be a perfect place to take in-calls. The going rate was $25 to $40. My clients ranged in age from the twenties to the seventies. The money helped me to get through this rough financial time. Denis was wary, not because of the sex, per se, but because of potential physical and legal dangers. Ours was an "open" relationship, based not on monogamy but rather on mutual respect and honesty. Indeed, during this period Denis was pursuing his own sexual proclivities.

I continued looking for a job, and by September I landed a position in the accounting department at Children's Hospital, but within several weeks I came down with hepatitis. My recovery took several months, but as an aftermath, I noticed that it took more energy for me to walk, especially inclined surfaces. This was a first indication of other long term problems down the road from STD exposures. I surmised that a few recent unsafe sexual encounters were the source of my exposure. I was weak and laid up for two months but Children's hospital graciously held my job, and I was able to resume work later that year.

27. MY NEW CAREER

One year after the purchase of our home on Alpine Terrace the balance owed on our contract of Sale was due and payable. I called my friend Don, and asked him to refer me to a realtor for help. He suggested two active gay realtors. One was an "older" realtor, Brad Lampley, and the other was a "younger" realtor, Paul Langley. We called Paul, and he told us what to do to save our investment in our home, and we proceeded to apply and qualify for a new mortgage.

Paul found out that I had a broker's license in Illinois and offered me a spot in his real estate company as a sales agent. I had vowed never to go back into real estate sales because of the uncertainty of a steady income. His offer presented me with a dilemma. My original reason for going into brokerage was to have an interesting career. My time in real estate had certainly been "interesting," but too often disheartening. I reconsidered, and I took the California brokers exam and joined Paul Langley and Co. whose office was at 25th and Clement in the outer Richmond district. I told Paul that I was earning money escorting and would need to continue that until I established myself with commission earnings. He agreed. I was now looking to cultivate real estate clients while still augmenting my income escorting.

One day late in 1971, I went on an outcall to meet a client at the Del Webb Townhouse complex at eleventh and Market Streets. There I met a man who seemed a bit reticent, and immediately proceeded to step out into the hall for a "breath of fresh air," when in rushed the vice squad to arrest me for prostitution. They hauled me off to the police station and booked me. I called Paul and he bailed me out with $500 cash that he kept for just such emergencies. I contacted an attorney who eventually reduced the charges to moral turpitude. My only fear was that this arrest would impair my real estate license. Luckily, about this time the state of California decoupled any arrests for moral turpitude, and they could no longer require the cancellation of my license. After that incident, I concentrated on selling real estate!

As I have revealed, Castro Street was exploding and there were new gay bars opening every few months. The old Irish and German haunts were being replaced at a remarkable pace. The momentum was unbelievable and the mystique of Castro Street as the coming gay mecca was obvious to me. The word was out throughout the Country that gay life was thriving in San Francisco. I called this new wave of activity to the attention of Paul Langley and proposed that he should have an office presence in this volatile and exciting neighborhood. About this time, I met a woman who mentioned that she was one of the heirs of the deceased owner of a corner commercial property at eighteenth and Castro. The property was a dilapidated building that housed an old-line drug store, in the process of closing its doors after 70 years in business. The upstairs was essentially vacant and in disrepair. She wanted her family to sell it and take the proceeds. I immediately told Paul that this would make a great place to have his office. Paul jumped in and negotiated with the owners and bought the building. The price was $400,000, and on this sale I earned my first big commission.

Paul went to work remodeling the entire building and the upstairs for offices. He moved his staff into this location in 1973. He was now in a great position to expand and further build up his company as a brokerage that catered to the newly arriving gay men flooding the neighborhood.

There existed a situation that many existing, old time residents were anxious to leave the city, because of the hippies encroaching from the Haight Ashbury and from blacks that had an increasing presence to the North in the Western Addition. This dynamic set the stage for some exciting new opportunities for gay men wanting to make the neighborhood their new home and we, as agents working for Paul Langley & Co. had access to eager clients who wanted to buy properties in the City.

28. GETAWAYS

As I started to make real estate sales, I met people who were having thoughts about an expanded social life outside the city. One of my clients suggested that we vacation in Palm Springs. We were told to stay at Dave's Villa Caprice in Cathedral City, so Denis and I took the bait. I fully remember the excitement of my first visit, stepping off the plane onto the tarmac at PSP just steps away from their new terminal. In those days, the Villa Caprice resort sent a driver to pick up guests arriving by plane. Richard Locke, an early seventies porn star who worked there as a masseur, picked me up.

One of the fashions in the early seventies was to wear floor length caftans, so Denis and I had our client friends in San Francisco create a matching pair for us to wear. The winter weather in Palm Springs was warm and sunny and provided a nice break from the cooler and rainy SF Winter weather. The grounds at the Villa were completely private, so that nudity was the norm. In both the public and private rooms and the tone was laid back sensual.

Our trips to Palm Springs were frequent in the early seventies but they tapered off when we found a country paradise closer to the City. While looking through an ad in the *Bay Area Reporter* one day, I noticed that a getaway group was being formed for a weekend in Sonoma County. It was at Wildwood Ranch above the Russian River in Guerneville, Ca.

Denis thought I should have some recreation time away from my hectic real estate life, so I signed up one day in 1973 for a weekend in the country.

Our travelling group met at The Round Up, a South of Market country and western bar on the corner of sixth and Folsom. Seven of us piled into a van and off we went up highway 101 to Guerneville, about 1½ hours' drive north of the city. The route took us passed vineyards and over several picturesque bridges. As we came closer to town the magnificent tall trees spurred by heavy seasonal rainfall began to dominate the scenery.

Downtown Guerneville was a one-street affair that reminded me of the Delavan, Wisconsin of my youth. In fact, the Russian River was similarly a summer escape popular with the blue-collar families of San Francisco, who wanted country relaxation from the City's chilly summer weather. These families had all the benefits of homes nestled in the trees, swimming and boating on the river, and room to roam around. It was great for city families with children. There were also quite a few resorts that catered to the weekend people from San Francisco.

Continuing my first visit to Wildwood, we drove through downtown and turned onto Old Cazadero Road which wound upward into the hills. We travelled past the Manzanita trees at the 600-foot level and ultimately to our destination, a compound 1,200 feet above the Russian River.

Nickolas was the owner of the Wildwood Ranch and he was developing the ranch as a gay getaway. I immediately fell in love with both the beauty of the spot and of the beauty of Nick's idea, which was to bring gay men together to relax, hike, sun and party in the country. Those first years were extremely informal. All the food we had was brought up for the weekend. We ate in the main house, usually 10 to 12 men in the beginning. We had only one option, which was to sleep in the bunkhouse, a building with beds in a communal setup. Later the owner would construct a rustic building that would feature tiny but private rooms.

A short walk on the grounds brought us to an absolutely beautiful spot overlooking the valley below, which we dubbed "Julie Andrews Point." At times in the summer the fog would roll in from the sea through the valley below and collect as a moving river of clouds below us. It was a stunning site, as we were high above the fog line. Heaven on earth!

As word got out about Wildwood, more and more San Francisco men became interested in the area around the Russian River. Prices of real estate were dirt cheap. The old blue collar families were all too glad to sell their houses that had served their purpose through the years. Properties could be purchased for very little, but they usually needed lots of repairs and upgrading. This was a mirror image of what was happening in San Francisco, where the white blue collar owners wanted out from their commitment to the city because of the changing demographics.

29. SETTLING IN –
SAN FRANCISCO IN THE 1970s

It became apparent that picking Buena Vista Hill for our residence was an extremely wise choice. The neighborhood was becoming a center of social change and of intense real estate activity. During this time, Denis was happily keeping a busy constructive life. He became involved in the burgeoning gay theater scene and extension of the gay freedom movement of the early seventies. Through his connection with the casts of these productions, he met Don Cavallo, who owned a popular restaurant called The Fickle Fox in the Mission District, at nineteenth and Valencia. Don immediately recognized that Denis was a talented, sensitive pianist who could accompany any singer and make them sound good, even great, when singing a song. He hired Denis to play weekend nights at the piano bar at the front of his busy restaurant. I would often go the Fickle Fox and join in with the raucous singing, drinking and carousing crowd. It was the place to be in the seventies. Around midnight I would often go on to other gay haunts South of Market.

"South of Market" was an area starting to become popular as another gay meeting scene. It would augment the Castro and eventually equal it in terms of the number of gay establishments. The scene was darker and more leather and fetish-oriented than the Castro, where the "Castro Clone" look of jeans and "T" shirts ruled.

SOMA began to sprout alternative sex clubs so guys could choose a place to express their personal sexual preferences, and allow them to experiment. Most of these new venues were owned by members of the gay community, who would rent or buy underused commercial spaces. These were often cheap hotels that were in disuse or vacant, but perfect to set up creative spaces to attract the late night and all night crowds. Cubicles, Fantasy Spaces, Glory Holes, dark and dimly lit corridors were all part of the scene. Lots of sex on the premises. In fact, that was the whole purpose.

One of the bars in SOMA was the Red Star Saloon. It was connected to the Barracks sex club, and patrons could go back and forth between the venues. Many of the bars played loose and easy with the rules of the ABC, the Alcohol Beverage Commission, that frowned on public venues where alcohol and sex were mixed. All in all, many of the places were wildly erotic bordering on the illegal. There was also action taking place outside on the streets after hours. This was the environment when the restaurant Hamburger Mary's opened at eleventh and Howard streets. It operated after the bars closed and on into the morning light. Often I would be ordering a Mary Burger sitting at the counter at 2 AM or later.

30. POLITICS – "HARVEY AND ANITA"

Harvey Milk opened a camera shop in the early seventies on Castro Street. He was living a hippy life in San Francisco after shunning a fast-paced financial career in New Your City. I became aware of Harvey through our common interest in promoting neighborhood development in the Castro and met with him to promote the area's businesses. Harvey and I and seven other concerned business people got together in 1971 to discuss an agenda. Harvey conducted the meeting and did most of the talking. He was *very* directed, and pushed his ideas above all others. I thought he was a prima donna because he was not interested in anyone else's ideas. Eventually he became more politically active, and soon he became a very high profile mover and shaker in the City pushing a more open acceptance to the new, active gay community. This thrust launched his political career that resulted in his being elected as a city supervisor.

One seminal event occurred in 1973 that indicates the growing influence of the gay community in San Francisco at that time, and by extension the rising power of Harvey Milk. It was an event that was given absolutely no publicity to the general public. The new Market Street subway was just completed and ready to start operations. The local gay community, exclusively, was invited to a kick off the open house to the new system. Two trains from the brand new rolling stock were parked in the Castro station and the Van Ness Avenue stations. That evening the trains ran back and forth between those stations. The train cars were dimly lit and drinks and grass

(M.J.) were part of the festivities in the cars. It was one big party. Obviously, the gay community now had enough pull with City Hall to get this perk. This was just one seminal event in the transition of power from the old guard to the gay, activist community.

But this new-found power had a price. By 1975 there was a national backlash to the burgeoning gay power emerging in major cities. A push against emerging gay rights was spearheaded by Anita Bryant, "the orange juice queen from Florida." The gay community responded with a "Save Our Human Rights" campaign which prompted the San Francisco community to get involved in opposition to her.

Our real estate office staff became radicalized, and we all took the train to Los Angeles to show our support at a fundraising concert at the Hollywood Bowl. The entertainment headlined Lily Tomlin, Richard Pryor and Bette Midler. The trip and concert were a resounding success. Richard Pryor in his opening act may not have realized the power of the audience and their intentions to push for gay equality, and he "lost it" at an early point in his routine. As I remember, he announced to the arena filled with gay people that he was disappointed in us, and that we should be working at least as hard for the equality and rights of black people. "Why don't you get off your asses" for black power he yelled. The audience was stunned.

Here is another person's account of Prior's outburst: "... *he invited the audience to kiss his black ass and told them about how, when he was young, he had enjoyed sucking somebody or other's dick.... If people were offended by his remarks, he said, 'I hope y'all get raped by black folks with clap.' Elsewhere, he boasted publicly of how much cocaine he had consumed: 'I could have bought Peru for all the shit I snorted.'"*

Pryor was a brilliant comedian known to be consumed by the cumulative injustices to the black community. However, at this venue he conveniently ignored the black community's general lack of support for the gay community. This incident illustrates the stupidity of making these remarks in front of a gay audience. Pryor's behavior that afternoon startled the entertainment industry and they took him to task, but he eventually recovered his moxie and went on to have a stellar career.

When Bette Midler who had heard his insults, came onstage for the second half of the show, the first thing she said was "he can kiss my big fat white ass," which brought the house down.

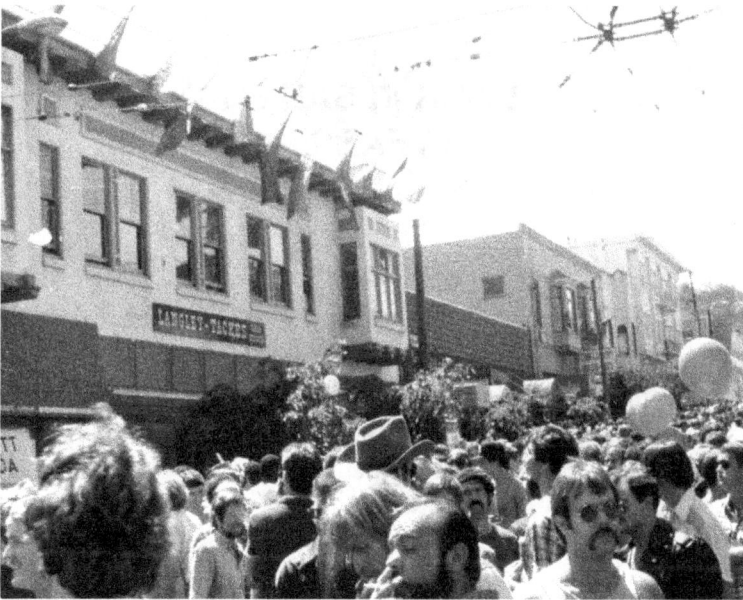

18th and Castro, San Francisco. A touch of partying outside my offices.

31. HIGH-FLYING IN SAN FRANCISCO
THE POWER YEARS – 1975-1980

Along with the influx of gay residents to San Francisco in the early 1970s, there was an influx of new money. Once sleepy neighborhoods like The Castro and Noe Valley were gentrified and quickly became a magnet for home buyers. Prices were affordable and down payments were low to the majority of gay men who had a job.

Paul Langley real estate agents were ready to blossom as neighborhood brokers and become part of the burgeoning transformation taking place in the City. The company name, PAUL LANGLEY & CO., was up on the side of the building at eighteenth and Castro for all to see. A number of new agents were recruited to join us in our second-floor offices. Paul Langley & Co. was flourishing, and so was I, with a decent flow of clients and commissions.

One of the first referrals I had was to lease a vacant apartment on Castro Street near Fourteenth Street. A young man named Dennis Peron contacted me and filled out an application. His references where not that strong, and when he became insistent, we approved him as tenant even though he gave the vibe that he thought we were discriminating against him. As it turned out he went on to be instrumental and very successful in the fight for liberalized law enforcement, and ultimately to achieve the legalization of medical and recreational Marijuana.

By the mid-1970s Paul Langley was burning out with the pressures of the business and the responsibility of managing the large agent staff. In mid-1975 Paul approached me with an offer to buy his brokerage business, because he trusted me and I had proved myself by applying myself diligently to my career.

This offer came to me out of the blue. I discussed this opportunity at length with Denis and we weighed what this might mean for our future. The responsibilities would be enormous. Would I be up to the challenge? It was one of those toss-of-the-coin yes or no life changing decisions. Part of me said no, because of my doubts about my ability to manage. Part of me said yes, remembering my father's extreme reluctance to take any chances at the height of the post World War II economic expansion. By becoming the owner and broker of this company I would be changing the course of my life.

My decision was to go ahead and purchase the brokerage business and hope for the best. It could be an opportunity to make some waves in my desire to help the gay rights movement, if it was successful. I felt that my involvement could become an aggressive instrument to tout the new era of gay power in the business and social communities. Paul provided me with several months of transitional training and paved the way for the staff to accept me as their new broker.

The next hectic months were a big challenge for me. I soon discovered that management of so many agents and staff became nerve wracking for me as well, so I hired a sales manager to take the brunt of operating, and handling day to day problems. Over the next few years I personally concentrated on planning further expansion and hiring, which in retrospect was a mistake. I had in mind a dramatic, but ultimately unrealistic expectation of substantial commission earnings from each agent that I hired, and thought that the increased agent output would justify more expansion.

Unfounded rumors that a rival Castro Street brokerage was going to open an Oakland location prompted me to open my second office, in a building that I purchased in the Lake Merritt neighborhood, a picturesque, hilly area near downtown Oakland. It was attracting lots of gay interest in the mid-70s.

Later I opened a third office in the upscale San Francisco Pacific Heights neighborhood, which gave the company a presence there and in the Upper Western Addition, which was also starting to be gentrified. The pace of growth and my belief that my staff of mainly inexperienced agents could start producing enough business gave me an initial headiness and euphoria.

In my heyday as a community realtor I was occupied with power lunches, frequent trips over the Bay Bridge to my Oakland office, and recognition in the San Francisco press as part of the new establishment. I embarked on an expensive expansion. About this time, Bill Beardemphal, the publisher of one of the local gay newspapers, the centrist *Sentinel*, asked me to write a column on real estate. In a gutsy mood I said yes. Bill thought a lot of me and my company. He was more business friendly than Harvey Milk and the *Bay Area Reporter* (BAR), which was the more politically correct gay paper of the era. In my *Sentinel* column, every two weeks, I sat down and wrote and shared tips that would be helpful to people wanting to own real estate.

Training and management development in my company, however, never became quite the success that I had hoped. As the decade progressed, my staff in three offices did grow to seventy-five. My three sales managers tried their hardest to get the sales staff to produce as per my projections, but unfortunately the staff couldn't deliver on these expectations.

My Castro office was known as a party place. Most of the staff was young and intimately involved in the swirl of nightlife and other distractions occurring in San Francisco, however, I was out of the loop on some things. It was many years later, that for example, that I found out that "Brownie Mary," a local who was known far and wide, was making her weekly Friday rounds in my office and taking orders for her notoriously good marijuana brownies. I would have happily purchased some!

As sales and commissions were coming in strong to the firm, I was able to purchase several apartment buildings in San Francisco. At the time, they could be purchased with very little cash down. My company office manager agreed to manage them for me. Unfortunately, these buildings had lots of deferred maintenance, but they increased nicely in value. Later, they became a source of operating funds that I used to continue the subsidy of my brokerage business.

In retrospect, if I had sold the brokerage business at that point at its high point, and focused on ownership of my properties I could have acquired a lot of wealth. The main problem was that I gave too much effort to expand the company, too fast, and without seasoned agents. This is all water under the bridge, and I have accepted the consequences, and have gone on with my life.

32. MY PERSONAL LIFE

While riding high on the expansion of Paul Langley and Company, my staff suggested that I should make some personal changes. They encouraged me to get rid of my car, a Gremlin, and buy one more worthy of a president of a corporation. I agreed, so I went down to the Jaguar dealership and plunked down $15,000, for a stunning new 1975 Jaguar SJC coupe. It was a beauty, cream colored with a black leather hard top and a slim maroon racing strip down the side. This was supposed to show the public that I had arrived.

Another opportunity immediately presented itself and set the stage for Denis and me to move into a more impressive home. A large Mediterranean house overlooking Dolores Park was a private, pocket listing of one of my sales associates.

We made an appointment to view the home. It was being occupied by an agent from another company who also wanted to buy it, but did not have the money. The day we had the inspection, he locked the door to the master bedroom suite so we could not get in. In addition, my listing agent disappeared during the process of the purchase, and to complicate matters more, another of my former agents put in a bid for the commission because she had had a previous listing on the property. This was getting dicey.

We loved the house and wanted it. To close the deal, I had to fly to Miami where I met with the owners directly and we signed the final papers.

When we bought the house, the rear yard was a mess and there was an ugly moat separating the house from the rest of the garden. We hired a landscape architect to produce a series of terraced decks in the rear with a Japanese Deco theme. There would be a sunken fire pit, a huge Jacuzzi and lots of palm and olive trees. After months of improvements we threw a large open house party for our friends and associates in the real estate business.

Soon after moving in, a wonderful cat appeared on our doorstep. Butchie soon joined us as the third member of our family, and was with us for the next eighteen years.

33. EXCESSES, FUN, EXPERIMENTATION

During this volatile period in the business world, I was continuing an active social life. There were many opportunities to party among the increasingly experimental lifestyles in the city. And I did. The South of Market bars and private clubs became more attractive to me as I took advantage of the specialized scenes in the City.

A typical night out might include a visit to the Stud, a classic devil-may-care bar with a serious group of revelers. The Stud had a small dance floor in the rear and a double bar that allowed everyone to see who was there and where I could take in all the action. The bar was always packed. My drink of choice was brandy and coffee. My other "upper of choice" was always those few tokes of marijuana. I would circulate and then take up a spot at the end of the bar near the dance floor. My buzz kicked in and I would occasionally step out onto the dance floor. One night in a haze I found myself dancing with a beautiful blond lady who suddenly transformed into my mother as a young woman. It was a miracle.

"Beautiful Bob" and I would commiserate at bars end, and drink our favorite drinks. Bob owned a used car lot by that name, at 1808 Market Street that was next door a sex club. This spot later became the site of the new the San Francisco Gay and Lesbian center.

After drinking at the Stud I usually moved on to after-hours clubs in SOMA or The Mission District, where an entirely new fantasy culture of bars and sex clubs was popping up. Drugs became a bigger ingredient as the seventies rolled on, but I rarely went beyond cannabis. Other men were much more daring. Some were experimenting with injectables. On occasion, I would accept cocaine from friends. Another popular drug was angel dust sprinkled on marijuana joint. This was an experiment that I soon realized was just too dangerous. Supposedly it was an animal tranquilizer. I had my one and only out-of-body experience when I smoked angel dust, and I found myself immobilized, yet floating freely above my actual self on the bed below. Luckily, I was with a sympathetic partner who carried me through the experience.

Poppers, of course, were ubiquitous because they heightened the sexual experience by creating a form of muscle relaxing euphoria. Poppers use started in the gay community way back in Chicago and continues to the present day.

One night at a SOMA club I met the Puerto Rican artist, Ramon Vidale, and we hit it off. After that I would talk with him periodically on Castro Street where he would perch himself on the sidewalk and paint scenes of ambiance in the Castro, and of the people inhabiting the neighborhood. He fancied himself a reincarnation of the essential "left bank," Parisian street artist, circa 1900. He had something there. Too bad he was not a trained artist, because if he had used more quality techniques, his works would now be more respected. Ramon was most prolific and he painted a huge number of canvasses. His works are now mainly held by private individuals, but so far have no known significant value.

Ramon said to me "Why don't I paint a portrait of you at your home. It could be clothed or nude." I took his suggestion and commissioned my infamous reclining nude-on-chaise-lounge painting. I chose the lounging pose I remembered from the classic cover photo of a young Truman Capote. We were both "ripped to the tits" while Ramon painted me. I display the portrait occasionally for private gatherings at my home. Ramon unfortunately, later died an early death from AIDS.

There were many other specialty bathhouses and clubs elsewhere in the city as the decade of the seventies rolled on. An old acquaintance from Wisconsin, Bob S. became my office receptionist and he introduced me to a notorious club in the basement of an historic Victorian in the Mission District. Also, coincidently or by design, Jose Serria, the first empress of San Francisco, lived in a flat upstairs. The entire block is now a historic district protected by the City. In the basement, the specialty was Hand Balling, FFA, and slings, and generally provided a venue for a real 'pig out' of excesses. As usual, my drugs of choice were alcohol, caffeine, poppers, and marijuana, and once they kicked in I was ready for action. People often asked me what I "was on" because I was so hyped up. I told them I was an easy high, which was true—a little bit of this and a little bit of that. They were impressed. Many of the other men, I suspected, were on heavy doses of more serious drugs in order to get into the mood so they could party hard and long. I am sure that my "moderation" in drug taking was the difference between their early deaths from HIV and my long life (also with HIV).

34. THE POLITICAL IMPACT OF HARVEY MILK

I was asked to speak at a local gathering of gay oriented businesses and I remember one occasion standing at the lectern giving my talk. Harvey Milk was sitting in the audience barely 15 feet in front of me. Milk clearly was not in the camp of business men and women selling real estate. His public stance was that realtors were capitalistic and destroying the outrageously affordable low rentals of his constituency.

Harvey was running for supervisor but so were several other gay candidates. I felt more comfortable with Rick Stokes, an attorney with more centrist ideas. As it turned out Harvey won the election at which point I was happy to support him so that he could garner enough power and votes to make a difference for the gay community. I recognized the effectiveness of Harvey's brash head-on assaults on the status quo. He was definitely in his element.

Harvey Milk was a huge figure in San Francisco during the 1970s. His asymmetrical brand of politics jolted the straight middle classes and fired up a groundswell to help homosexuals to gain more acceptance and power in the City. The Dan White assassination of mayor Moscone and Harvey Milk in the late seventies was sparked by Harvey's active disagreement with some of the old-line powers in San Francisco. The atmosphere in the city was polarized. Dan White was a supervisor who represented a working-class district in the Outer Mission. He was an ex fireman with a hot personality and he was not suited to public discourse, of to the supposed taunts that

Harvey sent his way. White became erratic. He resigned his supervisor's post and almost at once wanted to be reinstated. Mayor Moscone refused, most likely on the advice of Harvey Milk. This sparked White's bizarre mission to kill. He entered City Hall through an unlocked window, and shot Moscone and Milk. As a result of these murders, Dianne Feinstein became mayor, and eventually was elected to the United States senate.

I attended the protests that erupted after the murders and went right over to the Civic Plaza when the White Night riots took place. Police cars were burned and the doors to City Hall were smashed. That night, while I was at the Civic Center, there was a police action back at eighteenth and Castro, the very building where my offices were. The police had been fed up with the assaults on them at City Hall, and they proceeded to trash the Elephant Walk restaurant, which was directly below my offices upstairs. Luckily, we had no damage!

35. RETRENCHMENT – THE END OF AN ERA

In the late seventies, I began selling off the apartment buildings that I owned so that I could infuse operating cash into my business. It all came crashing down in 1980, when mortgage interest rates reached historic highs. By then my brokerage firm was losing $20,000 every month. Sales of real estate plummeted, I was losing money, I wanted out.

I bit the bullet and started to dismantle the company. It was a traumatic time and I do not revel in remembering all of the emotions and details of the machinations that it took to shutter my business.

The office I decided to close first was Oakland so I placed the building up for sale and all the agents were let go or integrated into my two remaining offices. The Union Street office at 2001 Union Street was the next to go. My lease was up, and the staff moved on to other venues. The last to go was my eighteenth and Castro office. Some people thought that I should stick it out but I terminated operations by the end of 1980. Tom Foster, my dedicated general manager, was instrumental in sorting out the main details of the dissolution. He was a gem, and worked for a year in my home to sort out the details of the closure.

The failure of my business coincided with the first public rumblings about a new, mysterious disease that was making gay men sick. In the summer of 1980, I had a bout of unexplained malaise and illness that kept me housebound for several months. I had no energy, no drive. After that my periods of health started to get shorter and shorter. All these complications, from the decline of my health to the failure of my business, created a massive fear in me. There was also a question of our severely lowered household income.

Denis remembers this period and says that I was in a lot of turmoil when my business started failing. He remembers thinking *"Well at least I've got a full-time job which is helping to bring in money. When you got ill, my first impression was that the rigors of shutting down business operations was affecting your health, so I was hoping the shutdown would be swift, so that your health would bounce back. I do recall thinking we would cope somehow, but we might have to sell our home to reduce expenses. Later on, I recall being immensely proud of you, when I realized you were making plans to pay back some of the money you owed Paul Langley, rather than simply declaring bankruptcy. By 1981 when we decided to put our home on the market, I recall pressuring you to accept a good but not great offer, because I was very concerned about your health, and felt we should get all these things behind us in order for you to regain peace."*

Denis and I had thought we would be living in that home "forever," but our attempts to find creative ways to afford it, and save our home came up against a dead end. We had to sell and move.

We rented a home on Roosevelt Way in the Corona Heights neighborhood for a few years, and then bought a modest home out in Glen Park, a short ride from The Castro.

36. HIV
"AIDS is a Heavy Meditation"

Having lost my company and my home all at once was the biggest blow of my life. The fact that Denis and I could only afford a home in the far reaches of San Francisco only heightened my depression. To make matters worse, I became very sick from out of nowhere. All of a sudden I felt helpless and I was sleeping poorly. I also was fatigued constantly, and on top of that I was losing weight but with no explanation. In fact, I became so ill that I was hospitalized. For the next four years, doctors failed to diagnose me, instead they credited my deteriorating health to stress. Then, once the HIV test first became available in 1985, I got tested. The results were HIV positive. My reaction was muted, because I had expected the worst leading up to the actual diagnosis. Several of my real estate agents were horrified by the spread of this disease, and thought they would escape San Francisco, return to their roots back home, and somehow cheat death. Well, that didn't work for them, it was too late. Another friend started going to Salt Lake City for his sexual liaisons, in the hope that the men there would not be as likely to have the disease. In his case, he was already infected, and he died shortly thereafter

My life was now in the hands of doctors who were searching and experimenting with many different kinds of treatments. The treatments at that time were purely speculative guesswork. Intensive biological work was being started by the medical community in order to understand the nature of the illness, so they could devise an effective protocol. Luckily, living in San Francisco at ground zero of this mystery epidemic, I had access to a variety of concerned medical and activist professionals who valiantly jumped in to find a cure.

During the 1980s I actively searched out a variety of alternative methods to stay alive. The abundant health resources in San Francisco were life savers. There was acupuncture and variations of massage. "Transfer Factor" was a regular injection therapy. Resources that I took advantage of included spiritualism, meditation and immune boosters of all sorts. I saw a Russian émigré to undergo hypnotism and enemas.

Marijuana was my lifesaver because it helped me both to relax and it would revitalize me. Marijuana took my mind off my malaise and got me out into stimulating social settings where I could meet new friends and engage in new activities. That's why I say marijuana saved my life, and why some people call me "a miracle" for surviving.

I did not have the experience of having huge numbers of close friends who were heavy drug users, and consequently did not have the additional traumas of seeing lots of friends dying close-up. I surmise that perhaps most of the infected men either had a stronger version of the virus, or they were not proactive enough to seek out the help that was being offered in our community. They did not survive long. I had myself to take care of, and I immediately pressed my health handlers to do something, anything to extend my life until there was a cure.

I was referred to a concerned doctor, Jon Kaiser, who picked up the treatment gauntlet early on in the epidemic. He managed to get me enrolled in alternative treatment groups. I had acupuncture, and although the positive results were not definitive, this and other treatments gave me a feeling that I would survive. There were body massages, and foot massages that were great relaxants. I was introduced to chi gung, a form of gentle exercise composed of movements that are repeated a number of times, often stretching the body, increasing fluid movement and building awareness of how the body moves through space. Medical doctors started to use transfer factor to help boost my immune system. I received regular, painful injections to my upper arms. These were all holding actions, but they gave me hope. All in all, it was dark time. The entire gay community continued to be gripped with fear.

In 1981, as I went into emotional lockdown, my sex and social life went on hold. The raucous gay life in San Francisco also came to a screeching halt and The Castro became a ghost town. Only when the Gay Games came to town in 1982 did it start to come alive again, because the games attracted a new crop of younger gay men. Many of the athletes and visitors were from areas of the country that had not yet been hit as hard with the plague. The offshoot of that influx for these games at Kezar stadium helped start a bit of life again in the city.

The 1980s clearly were a health nightmare for me. I call it my Death Decade. I had to force myself to get involved with constructive diversions that I could handle during periods that I felt relatively well. In the mid-eighties I was having night sweats. I continued to live under a general malaise caused by my HIV. However, I pushed myself to stay involved and productive in some way or other to get me through this period.

By the late eighties I gathered myself together and got involved in some limited real estate activity again. I was experiencing night and day sweats well into the 1990s. However, my health was stabilizing with the availability of more effective HIV medications.

Later, I became more confident and creative as I continued to pursue a positive health regimen. For example, I became more involved in designing and maintaining an elaborate garden. I walked the neighborhood streets for the Friends of the Urban Forest, to recruit sign-ups to plant trees in the sidewalks. I did a few brokerage stints for several of my old clients.

During this time, I continued going to the gym. This was a matter of health and body maintenance going all the way back to my late teens in Chicago. There was a remarkable gay gym on Hayes Street, just West of Davies Symphony Hall that was a dream place to work out.

I also about this time had more confidence to resume some of my South of Market safe sex encounters. It was most valuable to get out of the house daily and put myself into a distracting pleasant, cannabis high state of mind. One such event occurred at a South of Market sex club in the early nineties, when I "overdid" it.

It was the turn of the 21st century. San Francisco, the big City, continued to exert its charms, offering loads of opportunities for me to meet interesting people at bars, beaches, cafés and at the most creative sex clubs.

I'm having another night out at my favorite venue for sex. A hit or two of cannabis sets the mood. After checking in, I begin the parade through mazes, cubicles and ramps to access willing men. I am seeking Nirvana as are all the men here.

A little blue pill has helped me enhance my libido but unfortunately it also brings a smoky blue haze to my eyes in the half darkness. Feeling odd and woozy I sit down in the television room on a high wooden step.

Boing! I Pass out for a moment and fall forward and down onto the cement floor. There is a gash on my head above my eye but the fall brings me back to consciousness. Blood, then first aid and a shocked recovery, a drive home, then to sleep. It is a fair warning.

Never again, well hardly ever again, would I be seeking this kind of excess.

37. A NEW START – CAFÉ LIFE

Feeling devastated about the health limbo that I was in, I had to get out of the house or I would go crazy. One afternoon in 1985 I walked by the corner of Market and 16th Streets where I discovered a busy café. I had hardly paid attention or noticed it during my years of nighttime escapades doing the bar and sex club scene. I thought I would venture in and order a cup of coffee. This was the start of a long love affair with the Café Flore and a life that was to be my new alternative to nightlife in the bars.

Café Flore was a gathering place for a variety of offbeat and interesting laid back people. It was nothing like the frenetic bar scene where the patrons were hyped up and looking for sexual encounters. The café's patrons obviously had time on their hands to hang out. Many were jobless. Some were students and artists. They represented non-mainstream types as opposed to the sex and alcohol night people that I hung out with in the seventies. The vibes were beautiful there, with people who held a different attitude about life, and that intrigued me immensely.

The savvy Iranian owners of the Café Flore had a decisively alternative take on the local scene. For example, they had a seasonal habit of hanging a Christmas tree upside down from the vaulted ceiling inside. Perhaps a snide laugh at Christianity? Often the tree would stay up all year long. Eventually the tree was set up to rotate. Another hoot was the bathroom. It was tiny and unisexual, with an old basin and toilet that were squeezed into the wedge-shaped space. The walls and ceilings were used liberally to apply ever changing, witty graffiti. I had the nerve to add to it. I took a load of pictures of the interior, and made a huge collage with them that I may someday donate as a historical marker to recall those early days of the Café Flore.

I started to go to the Cafe almost every day. One or two hits of marijuana helped get me out of the house, and into the cafe where I could meditate, read and meet new people. It was not long before I latched on to some of the regulars. One day a group came bounding in apparently on some sort of high and very friendly, so I just hopped in with conversation. They turned out to be an immensely important core of people that helped ground me, heal me and make me feel alive again.

I met C.C. Fish, a lady who read tarot cards on the premises. There was Jeffrey "Dinesh" a sex-immersed hippy who was wildly sleeping around, but who also displayed an intense interest in classical music, eastern philosophy and the occult. Uri was an Israeli who was chilling out in San Francisco trying to find himself after spending time in India. John was a professorial gentleman who had a background in teaching and science. John-the-tall was a soft-spoken guy with a benevolent nature. He was a socialist/communist and he invited me to meet Angela Davis at an Oakland gathering where she was hosting a seminar. These were the people that became my closest friends.

Uri and I hit it off, partially because we really enjoyed our cannabis habit. Uri confessed to me that he started each day by getting high on cannabis. I would become a clever outward personality after smoking a few hits, after which I threw caution to the wind. Marijuana certainly allowed me to explore a part of my persona that alcohol never did. It allowed me to speak and interact with people without my usual reservations.

It's All Good! "The Cannabis experience has greatly improved my appreciation for art, a subject which I had never much appreciated before. The understanding of the intent of the artist which I can achieve when high sometimes carries over to when I'm down. This is one of man human frontiers which cannabis has helped me traverse." -CARL SAGAN

A whole new world opened for me. Because of my animated verboseness, the expressive use of my arms and face, Uri thought that I would be perfect to play the maid's part in Ionesco's *Bald Soprano*. He was planning a small production of the play that we could perform at performance spaces that were popping up all over the Market and Mission neighborhoods. My involvement in this production was a spur of the moment "Yes, let's do it."

After a few weeks of rehearsals and attempting to memorize my part it was clear that I could not memorize and remember my lines, nor become the flamboyant maid character when I was not terribly high. I withdrew. I will never forget that almost theatrical experience, and especially the delight and horror of almost having been an actress on a stage.

38. MY MOVE BACK TO THE CASTRO

After a few years, I became frustrated living in the boring Glen Park neighborhood and I started to drive around neighborhoods closer to the Castro to see where we might like to live. My excursions took me to the top of States Street where I saw a "For Sale" sign in front of a very impressive stand-alone three-unit building. It was an absolutely stunning location. Once the sale was completed we moved into the lower flat in 1987.

Our new home on States Street was situated on the side of a steep hill overlooking an idyllic canyon and the Vulcan stairway. Living there was a welcome relief to me and it was another thing that helped divert me from my health problems. Our new home was in a stunning setting, very much like a fairy tale Sausalito that was across the Golden Gate Bridge in Marin County. There were pine trees and palm trees right outside our windows. An original farm house was next door, and on the next lot down there was a home with a turret designed like a castle. We felt like we were in heaven in the heart of the City. Over the next nineteen years this was our home.

After we won the condo lottery in 2000 we converted to condominiums and we sold off the other two units. We moved into the top flat which had vaulted ceilings and even more spectacular views. I took charge of the garden below and did lots of planning, digging and planting. We had a pond with frogs, a Meyer lemon tree, a loquat tree and a fig tree. It was a true microclimate down at the lower end of our property. We really felt at home in this wonderful place!

39. PALM SPRINGS

Denis was retiring from his long-term teaching job and we had spent over 35 years having a rich life in San Francisco, but it was now time for a change, so we took a hard look at our future and discussed where we wanted to live the rest of our lives. Palm Springs had been a vacation destination as far back as the early 1970s and we were always ready to search out warmer climes, so we bought a condominium in Palm Springs in 2006 hoping to hold on to a pied d' Terre in San Francisco, but the San Francisco part soon became unrealistic.

We then turned our attention to finding the perfect house in Palm Springs. It took 6 months until we found a beautiful ranch home on the Tahquitz Creek golf course. We made the owners an offer they could not refuse and in 2007 we moved in. Our new home has beautiful vistas, and was designed by noted architect Donald Wexler. Although the home was a gem, we soon discovered that to make it fit our needs we needed to spend lots of money into making improvements. We tackled deferred maintenance and I took over the task of redesigning all the landscaping and supervising the renovations.

In 2009 Denis and I celebrated our 50 years together. A huge gathering of 100 of our friends was held at our home in April. In attendance was our friend Jose Sarria, the first empress of San Francisco. He led our mixed audience with a salute, and the entire crowd sang the rousing "God Save Us Nellie Queens." This song was an anthem from the early sixties in San Francisco, a time when Jose was instrumental in starting the gay resistance to the anti-gay police and the old-guard administration rampant at the time.

Denis and I have found new diversions in Palm Springs, and are delighted to have a myriad of choices it offers us. Denis has made contacts in the musical and theater world and we both have discovered new friends at a welcoming group of cafés that allow us to continue our love affair with daytime socializing.

In addition to café life, I started to attend a number of daytime resorts. There was a premier gay resort in Cathedral City called CCBC, the Cathedral City Boys Club. The grounds were as beautiful as the old Villa Caprice and is one of the most popular places in the Coachella Valley for gay men. They have a national clientele including lots of locals and guys from Los Angeles and San Francisco. I have had a great time there and met some most interesting people, some of whom have become longtime friends. (I had to stop going there when those incessant walks around the grounds started wearing me out!)

As the years of the 21st century unfold Denis and I have become fully attuned to the variety of opportunities in the Palm Springs area. There is substantial live theater, including music concerts. We have an international film festival, hip music festivals such as "Coachella" and many venues both high-end and low-down that juice the pot.

Palm Springs more recently has become attractive to hip young people from Los Angeles and coastal California. The venues in Palm Springs are finally catering to a younger demographic and have added a new vibrancy into the valley. We are seeing more diverse groups as well from Asia and Europe and Latin America. Mexican-Americans, of a new generation in particular, are playing an ever more important role enriching the Coachella valley.

Theater groups are in abundance. Many new residents have an illustrious background in the arts and professions. Arts and theater groups thrive, and there is often recruiting in Los Angeles of first-rate talent. Older people can indulge their fantasies and actually become active again as actors, producers and performers.

The Coachella and Stagecoach festivals have spurred development of youth-centric resorts, which have opened to energetic crowds coming here from the California coast and all over the country. Exclusively gay resorts remain a mainstay but now have been joined by lots of new and re-imagined resorts for mixed crowds. This new desert scene benefits us all, and we "locals" get the benefit of meeting and knowing a broad array of humanity.

I met my new, best friend, Richard, at Koffi café in 2007. As I was ordering my coffee, he buzzed by, bubbling with some light-hearted comments. We discovered that we had many of the same roots. Truly separated at the hip! Our paths never crossed until Palm Springs, but we both related to youthful times in Wisconsin and San Francisco. For ten years in San Francisco we lived only a block away from each other but never met. Comparing notes from those important years cements our relationship. We speak candidly, often in shorthand when we are together, but always with a basic love and understanding.

I have been a witness to the gay marriage of friends. I see new friends coming to the desert for a new life. I see older friends winding down their lives and disappearing from the scene. I see Mexican youth moving into the American middle class and becoming a strong backbone of life here in the valley.

Amen. Ah...Men

40. EPILOGUE – FATE AND TIMING
"Toss of the Coin" Milestones

I occasionally reflect on how specific decisions during my lifetime have changed the course of my life. My choice to stay at home through college, rather than accept the four-year scholarship at St. Mary's in San Antonio, Texas, paved the way for my move to Evanston and the opportunity to meet Denis, my life partner.

The Choice of San Francisco instead of Los Angeles certainly has meant an entirely different trajectory for me.

My decision to say Yes to purchase a real estate brokerage firm, instead of continuing as a lone agent, brought me into the powerful arena of gay San Francisco history.

These were the choices that, if I had taken another path, would have made for a very different life. I am glad that I made the decisions that I did, and I have never looked back with serious regrets. The future remains misty. I have lived a wonderful life with Denis and I am immensely grateful for the bit of luck that has helped me to live an interesting, insane, honest, yet balanced existence.

The milestones that have shaped my life remain important to me. Childhood guidelines such as those offered by my father to "never tell a lie" have served me well. Dad enlarged that by saying, "It is easier to keep your life in order because you don't have to remember what you said, just work from your honest heart." Brother John in high school boldly stated, "Live your life with moderation. Excess can lead to disaster. Get the most pleasure and satisfaction from a balanced life." and that advice has helped me stay grounded. Professor Mogilnitsky in college reminded me to "Stay current. Read periodicals of all sorts so you are prepared for the future."

My sacred triangle of the important things in life keeps evolving:

1. Sex and sensuality. Enjoy it to the fullest. God's gift. It now has a more measured role.

2. Real Estate. This is now relegated mostly to our home. My early fascination with real estate was important. It was something concrete, to be touched, lived in, savored and invested in. These days I have fresh impulses from time to time about having a second home in some exotic getaway place like Hawaii or the mountains above Palm Springs; perhaps in a university town like Santa Barbara or Redlands. But reality, financial and physical, says otherwise.

3. Marijuana. The engine of my soul. Now used diligently, and more sparingly. It has offered me courage to surmount my basic guarded and reluctant nature, and allowed me to project an air of confidence and conviviality. It also has helped distract me from years of pain and uncertainty while I adjusted my mind and body to the challenges of HIV.

I have mellowed. I read more, I party less. I stay current about movements affecting our very existence on the planet. I have finally come to have a more realistic view of the world, based on my experiences. I relate to others better.

Human nature can be highly unhinged, but awareness of what is happening around me places my life in more perspective. In many respects, I am still and again more of an observer, remembering my father's warning that there is danger in becoming too involved in pride, passion, and the pursuit of power.

PART THREE

EMOTIONAL HIGHS & LOWS
Flights of Fancy

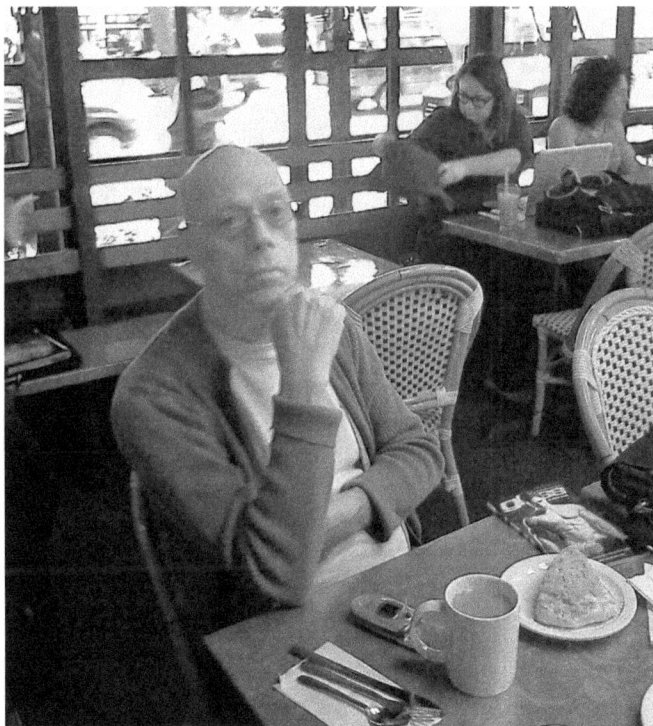

Rob at Café Flore, 1990s.

Emotional Musings
Reminiscing in Depth
Coming Out
HIV Challenges
Fear & Joy
Creative Spaces
Dada
Accommodation

41. INTRODUCTION TO THE DANCE

In Parts One and Two of my memoir I recount events of my life in a narrative style.

Part Three is more concerned with my flights of fancy, artistic and spiritual matters, especially my volatile emotional state in the 1980s and 1990s as it played itself out. Hope arose, and I regained some stability to my health.

Part Three showcases some of my letters, journals, and my whimsical poetry during that period.

Many of these exercises are a form of DADA, with wild shifts of tone, at times irrational, at times negative, yet all relevant to my mindset of the time. Some of my musings are experiences in the flesh; others are pure flights of imagination that reflect the joys and disappointments of the moment. Those reflections, happily enhanced by cannabis highs, enabled me to ponder in a deeper way the events happening around me, and I was released emotionally to notice interactions and meanings that I might otherwise have missed.

Some of the expositions are X-Rated, dream-like, and cut to the chase of my zestful sexual infatuation.

Part Four lightens up and recounts some of my most favorite things!

[Note: In the following selections, the texts of the 1979-96 letters, journals and poetry are set in Romanized (regular) print; and my 2016 reflections on these letters, journals and poetry are set in *italicized print*.]

42. CORRESPONDENCE WITH MY FAMILY

In the late seventies, I signed up to The Advocate Experience. It was a guided self-help retreat for gay men and women to help them cope with a number of challenging situations that they may have to face in a mostly heterosexual world. The Experience strongly recommended that we come out to our parents if we had not already done so. Dad was 74 and I was 42 in 1979, and as a prompt from The Advocate Experience I had the opportunity and motivation to finally, officially "Come Out" to my father.

As a result, I wrote my dad a long handwritten letter stating that I was gay. He, as well as my immediate family may have supposed it, but sexuality was never discussed in our family, so this letter was to make it "official." In re-reading my letter after many years I realize that I took the moderator's advice to heart and I fashioned a specific although a somewhat stultified and mundane piece.

January 22, 1979

Dear Dad,

I felt real good talking to you on the telephone in such a natural manner in December. I've felt in recent months that the time was growing near that it would be OK for me to tell you that I am gay and that I am living an extremely happy and rewarding life in San Francisco. The other thing that I want to tell you is that I love you, and always have, but circumstances have made it difficult for me to communicate this to you.

The third and most important thing to me now is to thank you and mom for everything you did that laid the foundation for me so I could be the complete, happy and successful person I am today. Somehow it has all come out perfectly. In case you had some doubts about the positive value of both of your contributions to my life, lay those doubts to rest, because I am now entering a period of my life in which I can now share all these good things that I've finally put together for myself, and which help me make life here on the West Coast fuller and more complete.

You have a lot to be proud of, and I realize now that it hasn't been easy, it never is, to accomplish anything good in life that is worthwhile.

I don't expect that this letter will necessarily make our relationship in the future any different, and I know that we are "coming from different places". When you have digested this letter and my thoughts I hope you can acknowledge me in any way that you feel comfortable. It can be short or long; letter or telephone, here or there, just so it is your honest reaction. That is all we have to live with. I am in the dark about your feelings and reactions and I can accept your reaction, whatever it is.

I'm happy to get this entire out to you; it's been a long time coming.

Your loving son, Bob.

P.S. Did you know people have called me "Rob" out here since 1970? Did you know that Denis and I are celebrating our 20th year together in April?

Here is my dad's response, a typical non-interfering reaction to my very personal, sexual disclosures.

January 30, 1979

Dear Rob,

It's been a long time since I wrote a letter. I was happy to hear from you. I liked the letter you wrote. I never knew that you felt that way about Clara and me. I sure wish Clara could have read the letter. That would have made her real happy. She was always concerned about you. She would always ask me "I wonder why Bob doesn't write or call." She thought about you a lot. It's too bad I lost her. We were getting along real well together.

Let's talk about the snow. I think I have seen more snow this year, and longer than ever before. They have to plow our home going out of our driveway. It's piling 8 feet high.

I have been feeling pretty good. I had the flu for about a week, that set me back a little. Now I have an irritation on my back side and itching like crazy. I called my two brothers and sister for the holidays. They are fairly well. John had a severe operation. He had plastic veins put into his legs. He is walking without his cane now. I called him about a week ago and told him about our snow. He laughed and said "you should see what we get" they hadn't been to church all of January.

Ed and Elsie Sanaghan are out in Arizona. I guess Eddie and Lori are having problems. So Elsie is going to straighten it out.

[My Aunt Elsie was an action oriented woman, much like grandpa Ascherl, unlike my mother who was more retiring like grandma Ascherl.]

[Brother] Tom and Patti are supposed to drive out to Arizona in February and they will drive Patti's folk's station wagon, and then fly back. Her folks flew out there some time back. Dianne, [a neighbor], had me over for dinner last week. She visits from time to time. So do some of my other neighbors. At one time I had 3 snow blowers in my garage.

I received an invite to my class reunion from Random Lake High School on the twenty forth of June. There are not many left anymore so they are combining a number of classes.

I am going up to Jerrys over the weekend. I'll have him make out my income tax forms. It looks like I am going to owe them a lot of money according to Tommy. I don't understand it because last year I got all the money back. I still haven't paid my doctor bills.

I guess this will be it for this time. Excuse the paper I am using. I was going to rewrite it on white paper but found it was too much work

From your Dad with love. Thomas N. Tackes

Reading my dad's response after all these years, I was reminded of how easily he brushed off the elements of my gay revelation. He switches gear and proceeds to write about things that for him were much more comfortable territory—the ins and outs of daily living. This was consistent with our family's history of avoiding talking about sex and matters of emotion during my growing up years.

In his letter, I was extremely moved by my dad's comments about Clara, my mother's sister, whom he married after my mother died. It was a reminder of how much she and

they thought that I had abandoned them. In a way I did. I had to get away from the mundanity of it all. On the other hand, I wish that there could have been discussions, not only of my situation, but also of Clara and Dad's hopes and dreams from their earlier years. There must have been plenty of excitement in Clara's life, and possibly even in my dad's life. But true to our family's Germanic traditions virtually no in depth discussions about hope and fears ever took place. My mother, Lily, and Dad's emotional lives remain an unspoken mystery to me. Dad hints very little of any introspection in his letter to me.

My uncle Art was another important family member. He was my confirmation sponsor. Arthur is my given 4th name. Art was an enigma and somewhat intimidating to me because of the intellectual challenges he posed. Art made it a point to take me under his wing, attempting to help me become more aware of the world, outside of our inwardly focused family. I did not "get it" until later in life.

Here is a letter from him long after I had moved to California. I had written to my uncle Art giving him an update on what was happening in my life. In response, he wrote me this letter. It provided me with an opportunity to relate to an important relative as an adult. Wow. I was blown away reading this again.

January 16, 1982

Dear Bob,

Janet and I got married on November 20th.

[Art was 64 years old and had been living with Janet for a while. Art was never married until later in his life. I occasionally wondered whether he might be gay, but apparently he was just unhappy with his life, partly due to frustrations about missing out on a top-notch education at IIT, the Illinois Institute of Technology.]

We are fairly happy and comfortable all things considered.

I wonder why you no longer keep in touch with us. You have always been in my thoughts a lot. I worry about your health and lifestyle. Let us know if you are O.K.

[Here is that same theme and concern that my aunt Clara had. Both she and Art were most probably aware that I was living the gay life in San Francisco. I now see that they really cared about me.]

Your father never seemed interested in keeping up occasional contacts. Janet and I at first tried to get him to go out to dinner with us. I tried inviting him after Clara died; he never returned any phone calls.

[Something obviously was grating my dad about Art. Strange, because during the 1930's my father treated Art, who was my mother's kid brother, to all kinds of special treats. My dad was a sports fan and often got Art tickets to prize fights, hockey and football games and the like. Later on, Art drifted from job to job and sometimes borrowed money from my mom, when there was very little income in our household. In the early 1940s Art entered the Seminary to become a priest. (The joy of every German Catholic mother was to have a priest in the family.) This was especially important to grandma Ascherl. Well, Art dropped out of the seminary. I remember in the late 1940s he was employed as a caretaker for our parish buildings. After that he moved from job to job as a machinist. He became a top-notch machinist but had a bit of a temper and would too often resign in a huff if the boss rubbed him the wrong way.]

Tommy [my brother] seems mighty angry about something- I don't recall ever being malicious. Jerry the same, he is completely gone as far as any remnant of relationship. Your mother was always my favorite sister. Please let me know if your father has changed addresses. Janet and I would visit him.

We keep busy with Janet's son and daughter and four grandchildren. Had a lovely Christmas. Today we are going to see the Phantom of the Opera at the Candlelight Playhouse. Yesterday it was the Adler Planetarium and the Beluga Whales.

I hope your physical and financial health is good.

As ever, Uncle Art

INCURSIONS INTO SELF-HELP:

After my health began to decline in the 1980s due to infection with HIV, in the late 80s and early 90s I was seeking more spiritual grounding to help me cope with my ongoing HIV health problems.

I signed up to the courses of The Rosicrucians in the 80s. Their initial study material was a comprehensive story of mankind, which to me was much more interesting and logical than the bible. The well-organized lesson guides initially made good sense as they provided a rational approach to life here and beyond. As the lessons became more serious I followed some of their more esoteric rituals just to see that if these symbolic acts would help me solve some of my problems. Eventually the rituals became too overbearing and I terminated my membership, but I was left feeling that the exercises had helped me to understand paradigms other than the Christian view of the world.

Likewise, I immersed myself in The Raelian movement. This discipline attracted my attention in the 1990s, and the studies were another source of solace. Raelians posited an alternative view of reality and of the world and it helped me cope. Their theme was that Homo sapiens were infused with intelligence not by "God" but by advanced creatures from another plane. Why not?

In 1996, I wrote my brother Jerry and summarized some of the specific actions I had taken to prolong my life, giving me hope to survive the ravages of HIV.

My brother Jerry and I have kept up an open line of communication through the years. Here are some excerpts from my 1994 and 1996 letters to Jerry.

January 2, 1994

Dear Jerry,

The last 2 years have been spent disengaging from my "over-involving, compulsive" personality tendencies, and I still have a long way to go.

I am definitely slowing up, and age and my immune system's inability to protect me from my particular genetic weaknesses have forced me to keep disengaging until I can experience a sense of peace and health.

Fighting disease, finding ways to avoid serious emotional and physical impairment continue to be overriding factors in my day to day life.

On an equally serious note, I want to thank you for acting as my conduit, as you see fit, to make decisions regarding Dad.

Please let me know what is on your mind from time to time regarding any family decisions you may not want to make on your own.

Rob

October 10, 1996

Dear Jerry,

Just a note to let you know what's been going on in my life these last few years. At the moment I am reveling in a 3-month improvement in the way I feel. It's the most reliable energy I have experienced in over 15 years.

Basically I've utilized at least 5 professionals to help me gain better health. Through my visionary M.D., Jon Kaiser, I have embarked on a combination protocol that includes additional herbal and nutritional substances and these things:

-Chiropractic

-Acupuncture and Herbal solutions

-Anti Virals (3TC and D4T). Light dosages.

-Return to a light sensible workout with weights (Hot tub reward afterward!)

-Physical Therapy, to get me prepared to add the antivirals that are supposed to attack my very high viral load and also to give me whatever support I've need to improve my state of mind. I have also done several sessions on dream analysis--it has been eye-opening.

So there, I think that's about it. Wish me luck. I would really like to have much of my old energy back again so I can be a more engaged, contributing member of our community.

I have tried to convey a little bit of my most recent health and life concerns. I am telling you because you understand. You are welcome to be the conduit to anyone in the Midwest who needs to know "how I am" these days. Thanks again for your visits out here and for your on-site Chicago responsibilities.

Best of love to you and Karyn.

Rob

43. MY JOURNALS

Here are some of my extremely personal experiences and reflections in the 1990s. The years 1991-1996 were a dark period in my life. They put my 1980s "death decade" into a slightly different perspective

SOME OF THEM ARE VERY DARK!

The 1990s matched and sometimes surpassed the 1980s. I was experiencing HIV side effects into their second decade, and they were making me weary and were dragging me down, body and soul.

But life went on, its highs and lows. I kept as busy as I could, and marijuana got me out of the house so I could interact with people. All the while I would increasingly turn introspective and would scribble down my thoughts. Some notes recounted the beautiful experiences; some were the ramblings of my innermost fears and disappointments.

There was the promise of some new experimental HIV medications, but truly effective ones were still a long way off.

I aimed to lift myself out of the funks that continued to affect my health. From my random notes and journal entries I see that I was experiencing a questioning period about my health, and was concerned about financial and social matters. Those problems were building, and I was losing my ability to get a positive meaning out life. These were the frustrations that caused me to look for change. Was the change a new place to live or was it a new way to look at life?

I was able to maneuver around this negativity by forays to the beaches, the cafes, the out of town resorts, the sex clubs and generally by getting out of the house and using cannabis to keep on truckin'. My creative impulses helped me a lot.

April 1991

> City of Night
> City of Light
> City of Right
> City of Fright
> City of Blight

Now and then I got into some heavy thoughts about culture, society, investments, politics, hypocrisy and sex.

April 26, 1991

> LIFE
> Time to change regimens
> Everything just came together
> New, better drugs
> I'm wondering now, how
> I'll use the energy

7/16/91

Sex, Real Estate and Holidays. Let's deal with "work" now. Should work be play alone? Or should work be something you casually do and throw off.

Career. Something you put your heart, your soul into. Recognized in the business world. Something you do for the money. Time. Lots and lots of time.

7/17/91

What will motivate me now? If I'm not motivated I'll be bored. There's a chance of creating something exciting for the neighborhood.

A salon? Free advice. Display for local artists. Music, real estate, visual art.

7/30/91

What do I like doing? Buying and selling real estate. What can I make money doing? How do I do it?

7/31/91

Are we at "What's it all about Alphie" time again? What to do. What to do. Actually I do more of same only at a better pace for me. Is this more or less? Figure it out.

8/5/91

Bennett! My all weather fairie. Bring me to the woods. Soothe me. Make me think good thoughts.

8/7/91

LANDS END
Wow! The fog dancing on the sand.
Sun playing peek-a-boo
Beautiful man pulling on his foreskin.
Dog's snout burying in the sand.
Lovers making love on the beach.
The surf, the rocks look as they've never looked before.

8/13/91

So Phillip thought I was a writer. I am of sorts, I said. Nothing published yet. I do have my artistic aspects, I told him. Where have we met? You look really familiar. See you around Phillip.

8/14/91

Jason, Will you be the first? I could, could you?

8/19/91

Flore and an Early Rain.
Well, well. The sky is falling. Finally! Drops,
Drops, drops against the tin corrugated ceilings.
Flore! Flore! I love you!
We're having fun with our own mother
Nature. We just love the
Masochism of it all, and her welcome
Sadism to us.
Plenty of upturned mouths here
today and smiles, little smiles of
happiness due to mother's help.
In the far corner I see a lithe student
with an etched look. So young,
so pure appearing.
His notebook and my notebook cross
paths near the epicenter of the Café,
and so esoteric is this latte afternoon!

8/20/91

America is the refinement of European Culture
America is the integration of non-European Cultures.
America is the broadening of all world culture,
Citizens, avail yourselves of this great new culture

8/22/91

Do something with my life and share what I've learned w/ someone.

8/27/91

Plenty of Violins. A quiet, grey Monday at the Café.
White "T" shirts. 3 white "T" shirts at one table

8/27/91

Wonder if they're frat men. Six and a half feet of brown hunks. Yellow, sweet yellow eaters. Another school year starting. Men in process. Tight young men. Confident in their meekness. Virgins all.

8/27/91

The Café is a place of mystery. Not knowing what comes next. Who will walk through that door? Who is outside, now? Mysterious danger, the café...

9/11/91

Boy! She sounded like M. Hillis. She sounded like a real interesting young man.

Margaret Hillis of the Chicago Symphony Orchestra Chorus. Low voice and all.

9/11/91

Fog. Too much Fog. For September that is. But you're going to lose it. September sun, come around soon.

9/12/91

> All these smooth young faces.
> Egos to match.
> "Smooth City"
> For an afternoon.

9/18/91

Oh! The shallow pursuits of youth. No! The serious pursuits of youth. Another one to have and be loved by. Someone to love, or control? Energies all consuming. The thrust of life.

10/6/91

Marijuana is so nice. Opens me up. Depth of vision. A man above myself. Those Levi cracks look more fabulous too!

10/7/91

> Bosom buddies, Bosom buddies.
> How does your garden grow!
> Marvelous tits to ponder and press
> I understand what is on your mind.

10/19/91

The smoothness of the skin sitting in here is now being matched by the fifties smoothness of the lady crooners. The Italian language being spoken at the next table is student Italian. A combo of classic youth and classy fifties lady crooners. All these things bring me along with them.

10/19/91

Best friends. How it shows! Friends arriving and embracing. That look in their eyes. The last sun is setting in the crook of the roof lines across the street. Each time I look up the sun is framed so beautifully by a very particular SF façade. Jazzy and Hot.

10/19/91

At the beach today
It was so wide today.
The surf was so kind. What a comfort zone!
Derrin you nasty boy. It's time, the first in a long time.

10/27/91

Hal, Hal, Hal. Where did you come from? Your realities clash with my expectation of reality. My ideas of long ago.

What a wonderful man. A common ground for us to explore. Fashion and life. Baseball! Pittsburg. Hetro/Homo. Sane thinking among the insane others.

What a look from you. What a mouth. May I spit in it Sir?

10/27/91

What's the difference between a seer and a fraud?
    A fraud is a luckier man.

10/27/91

These 3 guys are talking at the Lone Star. 40s somethings, honestly masculine. They're talking about a common acquaintance. *"I don't know what's going on with him"* said one. *"He's just an old queer"* said another. The third man says *"What he is, is a jaded New York Jewish-American princess."* Yah.

10/30/91

Mary Jane. What a great connector. Opens up the mind. Surprises me anyway. Insight, depth, creation. The world needs more of this.

11/4/91

Stephen, you crazy guy! Native, Greek. Born March, 1969. Natural Son. Dizzy S.F. queer. Work, school, jewelry, glamour, attention!
    What wild undiscovered beauty do I yet get to see?

11/24/91

The world of fashion and finance meet at the Care Flore
    Jocks mild and strong.
    Fun looking men weave their web for all.
    People. People.

11/6/91

The young and the beautiful at the Flore today. Sounds of Tinkling glasses. Sitting by bamboo. A Provincetown summer here. The City is going about its business in its typical mad fashion at 2PM, at the Flore on this summer-like day.

11/6/91

Sensible West Linn Complex. $630,000 5.6 GRM. Very Nice Condition. Hurry. Owner/Agent

An ad dreamed up to sell our Portland property.

11/13/91

I'm beginning to wonder whether I should leave the complexities of Real Estate behind me now. Living in the present is not always that easy for me. It's work, even for the Monks!

11/18/91

Well, I'm back in balance and feeling good. Went back on Nystatin today because of some lovely spots on my tongue. Looking forward to my formal retirement by 2/6/92, thanks partially to the U.S. Government. I'm done killing myself, I think.

11/24/91

Just what is happening with this Asian thing? Control, superiority complexes I guess. Sorta like the Germans.

11/24/91

Oh blue building. Blue building will you ever be mine?

How trendy can I be? Can we use River Hill to obtain you? Will it make any economic sense? I can dream can't I? Yes I can!

River Hill was a suburban Portland apartment complex that we owned and the blue building was "The Glass Staircase" a high rise on the edge of downtown Portland, and a purchase that slipped away from our grasp due to some Portland funny business.

12/2/91

Those are great glasses big boy. Something for a summer December afternoon you had earlier? So did I, on Polk Street at three in the afternoon.

So here we are, both writing. Me, about my thought processes, and he?

Suburban 60s, lesbian 80s. I am doing it today with my new, too new, goatee. Well I guess this is the therapy I can look forward to from now on.

12/4/91

Are there only three kinds of people in the world?
1. Organized and Logical
2. Organized and emotional
3. Disorganized and lucky (or unlucky). Or What.

12/7/91

Potential Ad in the SF Times

Business Relationships wanted for business man and prescient dreamer. I am looking for entrepreneurs with financial resources and concrete goals to improve the quality of life in San Francisco, I have cost effective ideas that can be placed into action. Private Sector. Think Tanks. Profit oriented solutions preferred. Will contribute cerebral and creative help to these enterprises. Ownership participation nice but not necessary. Let's do lunch! Call Rob.

12/8/91

Reflections of the last 3 days.

Vitamin B-12. Am I making a breakthrough to a more mature way of living? Or is this false euphoria because of the sublingual B-1?

Something is telling me to simplify my life to resolve the dangling disquieting events and constraints of many and recent years. Energy and ideas can now flow through me and offer new solutions to old problems. "Challenges," Denis says.

Do I have the resources, the energies yet? Something needs to change now in order to validate my very being.

Is all life chemical? Is a sense of completion and finality at hand that will allow me to create something more positive for myself and others? We'll see. I hope I am ready for the challenge. Can I trust myself enough to cast off my compulsions? Compulsions which make me a prisoner of myself. Am I my own helper? My own beacon of light along the way, or do I need something else? Mana Carlota sena!

12/8/91

Sunday. Café Soma.

I'm on my way to the Eagle bar to FLY. Leaving home, where the sun is streaming through the West windows. The birds are trying to come out early. I'm coming out very late.

I think I'm ready to jump across the barriers to a kinder me. Denis, can you come with me! Or shall we continue our separate paths with impunity. Just concentrate on the Joy we give each other. Being with you is a special experience that has for a long time given me the freedom to be who I want to be. This kind of stability no one has the right to expect in this life. But I have it. I hope to grow up very soon and then act.

12/8/91

Start asking around for a handyman/cleaner/secretary. Someone to help Denis and me handle our deep commitments.

12/11/91

What to do. What to do. Just when am I going to be able to commit myself? What will it take? How much more introspection is needed? I definitely would like a salon across from the Café Flore. Should I ever own another building again? Or would I rather play with people than figures?

I could do analysis work (consulting) with entrepreneurs with my inheritance from Dad, or at least use my excess energy to successfully pull off a profitable venture.

12/18/91

I met with Nate Fox in Hollywood, Florida; He is starting a series of neighborhood newspapers and planning a network of nationwide contributors to write articles of genuine interest with a twist of truth, something "not seen often enough in the usual general circulation paper."

He's married. (Divorced?). Ex-girlfriend died in the Cayman Islands. Has an inheritance. Wants me to write and submit articles about San Francisco's cultural scene. Nate reminded me that he is a "compulsive" too! And he needs to keep busy. He says he just doesn't do business with anyone he doesn't like or trust.

Nate was a gay "Player" in 1960s Evanston. Moved out of sight. He mentioned at a later date that he became hooked on drugs. Do not know for sure.

Friday Night November 13, 1992

A wonderful party at Glenn Halak's

He brought along his spellbinding oil painting of a desert road to paradise and the cosmos.

Dinner, old friends, new marvelous people. Lake County on a ranchette. Gary just back. Glenn silent. Richard beaming and smiling large on my immediate left.

William of Ireland on my right. Dan reverting as usual and the rest of us going along for the ride! JD is so well behaved tonight. Aaron is his usual mix of laid-back and animated.

January 19, 1992

A little political philosophy
   "Ultimate Democracy" is the cause of self-destruction of any human society. The Ultimate Democracy assumes that each and every person knows and can agree on what is "best" for society, when in fact each person knows what is best for themselves alone. Rtt

----

1/22/92

Fourteen dollars in my pocket. (Less one latte). The mail person was late again today. Her vehicle stood in the gutter facing as I left down States Street. Well at least I got my package off to Portland in the five O'clock box at the post office. Later at the Flore a table was free; however I almost did have to pay fourteen dollars for it. The boy was nice.

1/22/92

BIKES!
   Helmets are beginning to appear everywhere. This Act-Up crowd is challenging the motor vehicle scenario. Of course that $100 fine is pretty clear, isn't it? A little societal discipline isn't a bad idea from time to time. Those boys and girls on bikes look like the crowd in "Blade Runner" or "Brazil." The San Francisco streets are surreal, especially around 5:30 in the afternoon.

1/22/92

Evening at home after meeting Irish Terry at the 1808 Sex Club.

One drop of water on my outstretched hands. A drop? I asked, half saying, half expressing to the young Irish guy in front of me. Irish Terry travelling the globe, in glamour no doubt. He grabbed me and we talked some more. Irish Terry wanted to get into a booth. Well. He's now in the cage and I'm 3 feet away, stopped in my tracks by the oh so charming stranger. I may not ever come out of there. Terry's personality is now coming across at 100% effectiveness!!

I step in and he grabs my dick, I his balls. And we rock together. He pinches my left tit too hard and I move (groan) "Lighten Up." And grab one of his nice tight buns, reveling in the strength of the flesh.

I can't go on. The experience is peppered with light wonderful thoughts. We wash together and talk together. He's a traveler all around the world. Filming here, porn I presume. This little Irish lad did it all for me. Shall we meet at Noon at the Café?

1/26/92

Blue Monday at the Café. No energy. Had to force myself out this afternoon. Two tokes, a black currant tea and a wonderful warm very round scone. A friendly visitor too.

We're talking about Markey Mark and violence in Guerneville. What about that model in the Sentinel. Is it really the same guy (Walter) sitting next to me? Stage makeup? He shares my table now. A first I think. Yes, the day is definitely getting pinker.

2/17/92

Record the new tax basis of our buildings in Portland--River Hill and the Milwaukian.

2/17/92

The asses of life, each with their own statements to make. Clothed loose or clothed tight in the fashion of the day. How much more expressive they would be if all were unclothed, especially those loosely clothed.

2/18/92

I need some better grass.

3/6/92

Here are two flowing tributes to the Café Flore from a guy I met at the Café, Freeman, who saw me writing poetry. He sat down and blew me away with his colorful writing.

"CAFÉ FLORE
The San Francesco twilight crept up and dulled the colors of Café Flore.

People sat edged on chairs and benched under tilted umbrellas that nervously shimmered in the cool breeze.

The trumpet of a recording drifted out from the café into the courtyard and mixed with the chatter and laughs of the café goers."

"THE GAUZE CURTAIN
Inside the Flore reggae music pulsed in the air as the coffee machine shot steam into frothy cups of milk and java. The low murmur of post- work voices breathed into the café an atmosphere of spentness. The weekend was beginning as the clients eased themselves into relaxation."

4/15/92

Just what IS this daily stomach pain? My anxiety out of control? Talk to W. about this. Therapy? More meds?

4/17/92

Our 33rd anniversary. The wind is blowing and I'm in a relaxed mood. What does it all mean? 33? Is it a magic bullet through the door? What is on the other side? More beauty I hope. Dee and I have to slow down. Somehow I think that the fruits of our lifetimes could be immediately ahead. I hope so. Will it happen naturally or should we do something formal?

Let's pick up on our natural curiosity about the popular arts. Populist venues. Euro Disney would get us to Europe again, to our beloved friends Howard and Malcolm. Or perhaps we can do something populist, American over here. Sedona, Prescott and Flagstaff perhaps? Let's get together with our friends again.

4/30/92

The Methodist church across the street from the Café Flore was torched by a person who did not like the fact that gay oriented theater was being presented in the meeting room. 23 years later this triangular lot on Market Street was still a hole in the ground!

They're bulldozing our hole across the street. The tractor road has been established. I wonder if they are going to build soon, and what will go up. For that I have only the brightest of hopes. A hallowed corner should get its due.

4/30/92

I read today that the community is planting a flower and vegetable garden at the Noe/Market spot. Too bad they can't open it up visually so we can all enjoy the beauty. I guess the fence needs to stay put so people do not fall into the depression.

4/27/92

Freeman says LA will not, repeat not, present me with viable opportunities to mix and find new friends, on a casual or an intellectual basis. "You must join a club that specializes, to be taken in... Otherwise be prepared to be rejected, sometimes overtly, by locals"

Freeman says that the bite of the movie business is everywhere. Many people have trouble separating their business life from the rest of their lives, thereby making it "impossible" to "avoid these people every day." Ultimate Frustration. Unnatural?

5/12/92

A rant and wishful thinking about nirvana on earth.

File this one in Personal. I'm really, really sick of people. I'm going to go into selective seclusion. I want a place of my own, by myself. Warm nights, some quiet cafes. A few interesting acquaintances. No pressures, no one to cow-tow to. Ignore all who upset me. I've had enough upset.

Why not an indoor Faerie circle? Resorts are ok too, but with indoor amenities. Titillation, stimulation, but very carefully. What use is there? Someone who cares. Can I rely on anyone else? Maybe one. I just want to fade away at my own pace and in control. No requests from anyone, just my own initiatives. A formula for disaster?

5/12/92 Tuesday

"RCP." May be a droll designation, by today's standards anyway. Does this crowd have any humanity at all? Just who are they really mad at? Mommy, Daddy? Perhaps they were all molested as children. Perhaps they can sue the system for monetary damages. Perhaps they will then all individually and collectively shut up. I am secure in the Middle Class.

5/12/92

Guilt? No, I'm getting on with the rest of my life. Please lord god of hosts; give me the strength to proceed.

Tonight might be pussy night at the 1808. I've been happiest alone. Is there a clue, a problem, a solution?

5/12/92

Peace, that's all I want. Peace. No more of this noise. No more advantage being taken of me. I just want to be left alone. Withdraw into the woodwork. Come out when I want to come out. Peace and no worry. What will it take? Death? Perhaps a quiet spot alone, except that I do not want to be alone. I'd like to spend much of my time on Ocean Beach or perhaps in Hawaii, if it is not too hot there. How can I break free from all this oppressive shit? Maybe a room in a friendly house. Turn over my affairs and tune out.

5/13/92

For Charlie. "Darling, why don't you just do your clients while you are in the sling?"

5/19/92

Looking for solutions.

Glenn says. "Do the acupuncture-ortho trip. Explore other weak spots in my system and have Mark address the Whole: "Set up a reasonable time frame review. Assess the benefits vs the costs. Otherwise go on to another alternative healing technique." Have I found it?

5/26/92

Pheromones. Do healthy things, to and for myself now. Negotiate a price I can afford, after conferring with experienced specialized practitioners and inspirers. Body, mind, spirit, budget. Mix them all together and what do you get? Bibbley, bobbley, boo!

6/1/92

Jim K. says, the "Book of Miracles" is better than "Seth Speaks" He says" Miracles" will help me put your life in wonderful order and balance."

6/2/92

Be myself, but don't get so ripped amongst the "general public."

6/12/92

I think we should sell River Hill. Become more liquid. Be able to take advantage of opportunities closer to SF which is our spiritual home now.

7/2/92

Isn't it about time that I find some more mature people to relate with?

The younger you are, the easier it is to be beautiful!

A tall man with the tight black Levis just walked in. It's the nice guy from the Oyster bar. Too bad he didn't see me. "You're sitting on my hand," Mark discretely sneered at me...

7/29/92

Oh what
Oh how
Oh where
Oh when
Oh please!

8/18/92

Blank Mind?
Focused Mind.
Let the rest of the world go bye.
Get involved

8/18/92

Why do I need to protect myself so much? Why am I so unnerved by the unexpected? Do I really need to handle everything well? What is it about my gut that makes me cower in fear? Aim to lighten up, that's it! Loosen up fuck up, so wakeup.

8/19/92

Those big brown eyes. They're sparkling huge in my face for the millisecond that our consciences meet.

8/22/92

Valter, crazy Valter. You have stood me up! Please come! We have so much to talk about. A little MJ and the right vibes go a long way. I'm looking forward to your prescience.

August, 1992.

Re: AIDS

   Per John James. Dr. Stephen Folensbee, expert on AIDS. Call him for a second opinion. (John thinks AZT is good enough for continuing use.) I am afraid of the side effects.

8/24/92

From the New Testament; "Matthew and John"

   OK young ones. Come on to me of your own free will and happiness. Make me happy too.

9/1/92

Dan. Dannie. Do I Dare?
There's something innocent about you. All that raging Charm!
You hypnotize me when you speak on.
Thanks for peeling away your succulent layers for me (to taste).

9/2/92

What is this thing called Café?
People come and people go.
People interact and don't interact.
All these personalities.
Our own little biosphere.

10/16/92

What truism can I shout? The old mold must be finished, very soon.
I hope I'm up for the next layer of this cake.

11/8/92

At Land's End last Sunday, and as I walked nude down the sandy strip.
A man appeared and he must have liked what he saw, or am I being too
presumptuous? Jim said a nice hello on this way to the water's edge. He looks
like he's really enjoying life. Seems ripped and happy. Lots of extra time on his
hands and he spends it well. Can I take a lesson from this?

11/9/92

At the Cafe again.

How wonderfully weird this multilayered menu that we have to pick from. To look or not to look. A variance of seconds can make all the difference while searching for a friend, or meeting a new friend. Shall I bounce with the music too? Well, just getting ready to "shake it."

11/16/92

Heuta Est. (oy!)
What does it mean?
Who am I?
Where am I at
The Cafe Flore, of course!

12/30/92

Freeman is the mystery composer of the previous florid account about the elegance of the Café Flore.

Freeman, you should publish that poem. It will stand on its own. Especially with the West Coast's artistic crowd. Is there an intellectual magazine in which you could get some important attention?

The poem's fluency hit me between the eyes throughout. I identify with the situations you describe. You write extremely well and the diversity of your points is presented to the readers' delight.

Yes, I do want to talk with you about your writing. What else do you have? Are you publishing a book? Tell me sometime soon.

1/7/93

Poop poop-edoo! Good jazz. Background drums coming from the other room. I'm filtering the music through this steamy, late January afternoon. It reminds me of the 70s. Great Jazz! Rain for days.

1/7/93

Santa Monica. Where could I become just a beach bum? Cozy little apartment not far from the beach and boardwalk, and very quiet. Lots of good guys are there and I am sure they are relaxing in the Cafes. A slower life for me. Denis can come down when he's in the mood. EZ drive to Palm Spring too, and Oceanside. Sort of Rob's heaven. Blue collar intellectuals as well as others. So easy to fart around with. Some warm nights. Easier winters. Sounds good to me. How about later in '93?

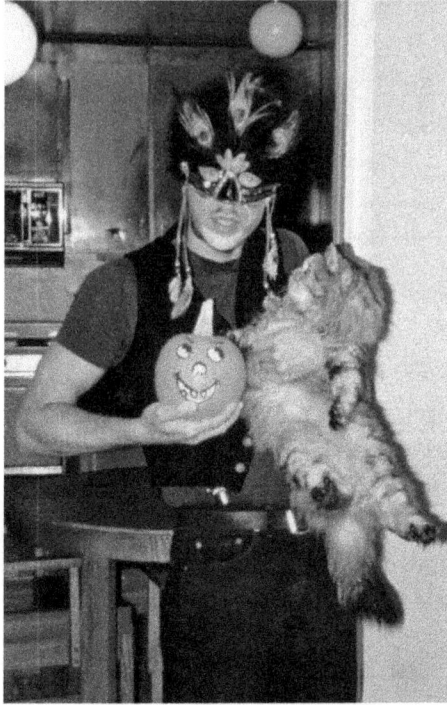

Halloween with Butchie, 1990s.

1/8/93

Oh why are we so uptight? What is it about our sacred bodies? Why can't we share them more easily? Perhaps it's more because our naked minds come to silly conclusions. After all, we all have something in common.

3/30/93

It's time to get old-school items taken care of. What new stuff will I be able to carry on with that will make me happier? I need to be easier with myself with the help of my friends. Calm between the excitements.

4/14/93

What is this pain in my groin and in my lower back? Had a good workout yesterday. I first felt the pain after coming out of the Hot Tub and while I was toweling myself dry. Most surprising. Anyway, let's see if I can give myself a tension rest over the next 14 days.

5/3/93

Musings on selling our Portland properties and dialing down on stress, caused by the angst of ownership. After Palm Springs. During my leg pain.

Sell our properties if possible. If we keep the Milwaukian pull back on rent increases and turnovers. Get rid of River Hill in 1993 if at all possible.

Simplify my fund investing approaches. Take more vacations from owning volatile funds.

5/10/93

At Flore.

Popping my meds down my gullet with my latte. I guess it's safe. I'm here in paradise so the results should be fine. Try to relax Rob, and enjoy your space.

5/10/93

Some milder form of mind therapy by Gary, along with some more physical massage would be a good mix for me to explore now. "Breathe honey; relax honey, for starter's honey."

6/4/93

Juan says: *See a good masseur for my Sciatica. Try creative, effective acupressure.*

6/20/93

Picture perfect me groping with my new limitations. Fitting in new situations. Slower ones, more sensuous if at all possible.

7/7/93

Is "Eros" open tonight? They don't have a shower there and the hot tub is grungy. Not many sex clubs have showers these days in SF. The plumbing is expensive.

9/20/93

Noticed on the john wall at SOMA Café. "When in doubt, smile and nod."

(*I feel a Hillary moment!*)

11/1/93

Have I run out of poetry or out of poetry time? Is poetry a chance to escape from time reality? I will write poetry more often. What a great antidote to problems with time.

11/1/93

Days are getting shorter—the time of year that I generally regret. This year however, I think I will have perpetual warmth through the otherwise dark season. My life is falling into place. At least this past week it has. Stability, order, sober evaluations, reconsiderations of life and the "doings" of my life. I hope I can reflect along with Denis and we can enjoy these changes together. Control is at hand. I feel it. Time to simplify and tie up my remaining loose ends. Time to relish and enjoy the process of quality living.

12/3/93

Reflections about my brother Tom. He was having health problems and subsequently died young.

Tom. How come you got so fat? Hope you see your sons grow up. They'll take care of you real well. I sure hope they go to college and travel and get to know more about the USA. I think it's time you move to Tucson. Life will be easier for you and Patti.

3/8/94

At Jumpin' Java - at Noe and Henry streets

1960s stream of consciousness music playing. Marvin Gaye. Place is full. Quieter than usual. Student and artists; Calmer, Straighter. Sade'

The Black boy/man to my left is writing a letter or doodling. Small squiggles in block penmanship. He starts at the upper right of the page and writes down in column of figures no larger than the "a" in figures. He stops to think. It must be a letter.

A young student roller bladed in, and just roller bladed out with his coffee to go. Oh yes, we're having August SF weather this afternoon. Thick and grey fog rolling in. Coming in dramatically over Twin Peaks. The air is pleasantly chilled.

3/8/94

More Jumpin' Java

And on my right is a long haired, young, exotic guy. He's smooth and his skin is a bone white. His art books and lesson assignment sheets bristle and blow with each opening and closing of the café's huge front door. It's a large studious crowd. Midterms are here. Coffees to go while walking home are popular. My berry scone was graciously cut in half, heated and served to me with butter. I ate it all. Meaningful cappuccinos here too. The best soy lattes in the City. Simultaneously peaceful and exciting--the space in here.

4/5/94

Is this it? Actually my mind's needs and my physical needs are quite different. Really, how worthwhile is spending 30-40 hours a week to make $20,000 extra each year. What would I do with 30 hours extra each week? Think about it and report back.

5/1/94

May Day

Rob. Should I forsake driving life efforts to "make it" of should I "Keep Pushing" to get closer to financial security as needed? Or neither.

5/13/94

On the wall of SOMA Café.
"SubLIME IS GAY"

6/2/94

Well here I am sitting again at the café Flore. Wondering whether I'll get my act together, or whether I'm going to go to pot. I'm removed from the scene more and more. But the power is still there because of my awareness of the interesting acts going on. Awareness. The power to relax and be at ease with yourself. Oh, to sustain such a tradition always.

6/20/94

Better figure out soon whether to retire from active investing and reach enlightenment on a tight budget. Or to continue my investment time and risk losing everything.

I was "day trading" at this point. Even rented a space in Loretta Young's mother's house in West Hollywood for a month's stay. Requested a separate phone line to conduct my fund trading. How's that for driven?

6/28/94

I wonder if it isn't time to retire. See what "T Bills" can earn me and have Denis cover the rest. Or find a less expensive place to live. Try to be creative. Ask Denis' opinion.

7/8/94

"Soma" Café. Ruminations on Rob's investment portfolio mix.

I am becoming obsessed with financial matters and looking more and more at wild, perhaps unaffordable real estate purchases. During the late nineties, we made offers on some very creative income properties that would have accommodated our living needs as well as provided income. None of these purchases were completed, partly because we were afraid we would be stretching our financial limits. In hindsight, they would have been smart moves to make.

8/26/94

It's about time to reduce my working hours to gain some more peace.
    Increase Zoloft to 50mg, every day.

While working with a social psychiatrist over a year or so, I tried three or four of the latest anti-depressants. None of them worked without annoying side effects, so I stopped taking them.

8/27/94

Well, today I rise from the depths of bedtime dreams, no nightmares, no aches and pains. Traded well. A short viewing with Debra then lunch. Shower and off to my M.D. I'm OK. Sure!

9/9/94

Am I old fashioned? Well today I dropped by Outer Haight Street. The current scene here has been called "cosmopolitan". But it's more white trash cosmopolitan.

9/16/94

Catch a falling star and put it in your weed pipe. All our 1950s history is being rejuggled by professionals. Historical perspective is nothing but one or more person's personal beliefs about what went on. Those personal realities suddenly make up society's ideas about how the world goes round. It's not Aristotle's logic.

9/28/94

Sitting in my car is almost like sitting in the café. The sun is streaming down on to my left front torso. I am waiting for Howard who is in the Hayes Street Gym. We are going to the Folsom Fair. Have the feeling we're going to have a real good time. (We did!)

11/5/94

What do I want now? I'd say more days off, mentally off.

What then? Things of the mind? Religion? Tai-Chi?

How about peace alone, or in small interesting, loving groups. And freedom to be warm in the winter.

Oh the Café life. That's it! Here and there.

11/9/94

Just had my first three-way conversation in some time. Glen, John and me.

A lot is going on, on the planet earth. We are talking collectively about a revolution. Blabbing about, screaming about, exposing, arguing, teaching, warning, understanding. Wonder if I will have long-conquered my battered immune system. Reality.

11/11/94

Soon the changes will be made. I feel it. I can live on a lot less income.

1/2/95

I've taken care of my life now, so let's get on with more of the pleasures. I need to be true to myself and I need to do that, here.

1/5/95

Christianity is all about intimate relationships. One that we have with ourselves, and one with others.

6/23/95

A Dream.

   Who did I notice along the Way in this night's dream? Remembrance.
   Mom, curiously enough. Dad, near and next to last. Young and sexy.
   Much earlier: Cousins, 2nd cousins, business associates, devilish guardian angels, stereotypes in a grand dark-light melodrama.
   Butchie, our cat. Financial security attained. To experience all this and then to start over with full knowledge and feeling for the past.
   Lots of love. Sexual understanding. No active deception in the final run-through.
   Total Recall! A chance meeting, a revisiting, a sexual climax. Germanic lust. Warm weather. Letters from Denis. Jesus, though not Paul.

6/25/95

What is worthwhile? Awareness of everything that isn't worthwhile.
   Freedom to be responsible. Respect for people along the way.
   Final realization and success at attaining a personal goal.
   Wild crescendo at the end of a journey.
   A simple, clean awakening heralded in the night.

6/25/95

TO DO:
Write a book of Political philosophy and Practical Action.
Ustinov's "One World," a myth or a possibility?
Point out an action structure that works.
Separate the individual's powers, not the governing powers.
Use the best practical solutions, the most balanced. Be a realistic day-to-day genius.
Ideally, elected politicians would rally the voters to support the best, realistic programs.
Try again, then try again with change.

7/3/95

What a depressing day, week, month. Poor health has become real for me. Wonder if I can ever get back to good health. Is it time for a change in my lifestyle. Maybe we should take a year off together.

Reconsider our lifestyle and emotional and physical needs. Financial realities. Better use of our thoughts, time, efforts, work, play. Redefine them.

8/30/95

Café Flore.
Klompin along with the horses. 3:35 PM the Kar-Mi clock says.
Horny men everywhere, young and old. Lascivious men wanting other men, wanting to be loved. The sooner we get some orgasm maker for the whole populace, the better. Now classical music is noticed, playing in the grand vocal style. It pervades this interior space. It all helps.

11/1/95

Get outside, get out, and get out Rob. Remember Chicago as a kid? I went to all of the museums, especially the popular cultural presentations in the outdoors.

12/26/95

Will my health hold long enough for me to make plans? What will I plan out for the next 5-7 years?

April 20, 1996

Trying to stave off a potentially upset stomach. Double soy latte, it's sorta weak. Me, sorta weak. What does my house hold for the rest of the century? Some ideas please Mr. Victor.

December 26, 1996

Café Flore. With this crowd today one must be a little curt. CDs are hung on the upside down Christmas tree this year. Very "Now." The tree is more discreet too, non-rotating. So continental. Nice! I wonder if Fort Lauderdale in the winter would be diverting enough. One can always try South Beach. Some future time. Build it into the Budget.

----

44. MY DREAMS & FLIGHTS OF FANCY

An XX-Rated Dream

A Dream Epiphany and a full case for chucking sexual repression and going for full sensuality.

Dear "Rob,"

From approximately 5:05 AM to 6:50 AM I had this fabulous semi-awake <u>dream</u>. Earlier I had a hard time fully sleeping, was "warm" and was experiencing one of the most annoying, deadening peripheral neuropathy pains--ever. Took a cup of breathe easy tea, watched TV, mostly Bloomberg market early results, and the Colorado high school terror incident.

I was in the usual over-my-head work situation. Working with computer associates (all men), who were much more astute and knowledgeable than I was. They seemed to be unusually adept and more free-thinking than the usual business associates of my past. At least that's how I perceived them. Various tasks, new equipment, new challenges for them and me, except that I really didn't think I could handle the technical challenges. There were different rooms, different colleagues, and different desks for me, and different changes happening all the time.

I decided that I had to escape, and found myself in an entirely new set of situations after my desk was destroyed with my basic life/work folders and 5 swimsuits. Lost when a building next door blew up and was now just a large lake.

I started meeting all sorts of adept, naked people as I left the old destroyed haunts. The crowd was racially, sexually, physically and preferentially incredibly talented in the variety of their sexual interests. They projected who they were and what they wanted!

I approached them individually, hesitant only slightly at first, and interacted with them. The first men were Asian and Japanese. Each person was displaying his own special self. One had a huge wide dick, one had a huge asshole, showing it to me while on his back and signaling for me to fuck him completely. I indicated my inability to get it hard and fulfill his first choice, so he offered me other options which I took.

Other scenarios, tableaus if you will, presented themselves. The men appearing were even more varied and specialized. Some were visually outrageous, especially in dress. One had a beautiful body and a smallish dick, but to entice me he immediately slapped on a huge dick to complement his large balls. He was administered to by others in the group. I immediately went down on his huge cock and took it all. Others took me from behind when they realized that I was very special.

Sensations of oral and anal sex entered my body. I shared fully with the other men, my physical needs, offerings, as well as other aspects of my reality. They appreciated me as much as I appreciated them. We parted at the end, knowing there would be more love, interaction and life for us all in the future, together.

There were no problems that seemed not to be able to be solved, understood, or be helpful for me. My problems were mostly mundane compared to the ecstasies we had experienced together. They helped me, and to cap my afternoon shared a sandwich/pasta with me before their 6PM closing. They gave me a communicating pair of glasses so I could ask an assistant where my car was parked. I felt reasonably sure of the future because I was only 5 blocks from home. We shared experiences of my rubber tooth which was disrupted by my sucking such large dicks. My $1,515 new front root canal impressed them and they related to it.

All this was enhanced with sights; sounds, full color, and full sensation so I chose to extend it, and then end it.

FINI.

This is the end of a snapshot of one intense five-year period in my life, and my ongoing quest for health and for direction. The next five years will bring me more angst but also more success in stabilizing my health. After 2001, I benefit from a four-drug HARP treatment that will keep my HIV Markers in an undetectable range.

After using the HARP medications my viral load became undetectable and remains so. There are downsides however, because long term use does cause ongoing side effects to many of my crucial organs, including the fact that I have lost my neat and trim waistline! Now I only have to worry about old age.

Still, I am glad to be alive!

Flights of Fancy

From time to time I would feel the urge to romanticize my experiences and convert my feelings into a more structured form. Here is some of my "Poetry."

Bad Boy Beach

At Land's End, San Francisco

I just went to heaven. I was in heaven and didn't have to die first.

We're all here cavorting with the boulders and outcroppings. What a joy to have the pleasure of their company. They have waited for us a long time.

Seagulls are dancing a ballet for me over the sea. Swinging and swaying with their great natural choreography.

Everyone on the beach is cleansed and we all feel very good indeed.

In this Natural Theater I sense that I am at the bottom of a 40 foot wide canyon above me. The view becomes a huge, leaning clay bas relief of "Dick Hotproud"...and me.

Looking up once more to the top of the canyon I see a shrine waving in the breeze. It is of golden reeds and Egyptian fans in all their natural glory. The rock canyon is protecting them on three sides. God and a few commandments shine from a plaque on the cliff behind.

Then the men. Many men. Fleshed out men with beautiful torso equipment. All Stars!

I continue-- center of my own elevated stage. Facing the ocean and the men.

My promontory dais lets me compete and give pleasure out here on this heavenly plain.

Jesus continues to wink at me from the face of the large sexy man of clay above me.

What a day.

San Francisco Metaphor

Where else on the planet Earth attracts like San Francisco. Young people from around the world come to the Cafe City. To live to work and to communicate their 21st century ideas.

What freedom and what beauty. Something's up with Mother Nature and we know what it is.

So easy to get around. The power points are here many agree. (Those who are here do agree.)

Multiple cultures whiff and waft around town. What a place to impregnate and procreate and bring birth to different ideas, the best ideas. No mere flesh, but the flesh made word.

This is a workshop for all here to test out our 21st century lives.

I believe at least we are ready to get smart on this planet. All those channels. Fabulous.

Intellectual property disseminated to the world. First here in the flesh, then as gossip to feed our revisionary ideas into the global consciousness. Invisible conversation and truly audible oceans of gossip

And *voila!*

The connections are made.

Café Generations

Old Queene! Actually he's pretty hot. Certainly well-traveled.

The "Dane and Swede" are 20 years apart but are achieving their sense of community here in front of my eyes.

It takes some strong initiatives and charm on OQ's part. He's turned on by the young Swede.

The Swede has plain young-boy qualities when his face is in repose. But oh! When he starts talking his animated face alone would propel him into Tom Cruisian roles in films. (This scene has strong desire and strong receptivity working.)

Working Class

We were working middle class.

It's very clear now. This is the best '90's way to describe my upbringing to young generations. Education was considered very important, especially a High School diploma.

I went to college. My Bachelor of Science got me out of the working class. Or did it?

Amazing how that B.S. was only the first crack in the door opening. It took me eventually into a world of self-exploration, sexual freedom, and to my ultimate self-realization.

What Now? Am I a little bored? Can this mean I'm ready to do something more important with my life! Scary. Yet...

Stay tuned.

Well Denis, can we talk? How can we start having a more normal life together? We should spend a lot more time creating some new places, where we can share some fine time.

Where-Oh Where can we go to start spending some more of our time together?

Or, Near a Campus! Warm climate in winters.

Maybe a real In-Center-City c o n d o, n e a r theater, p u b l i c events, and with warm weather in winter!

Must Speak English

Miami. Sydney. L.A.?? Melbourne, Brisbane?

August-End Musings

Gotta get a camera and start "taking" San Francisco.
Start with the "Amazing Cleaners" building
down on Laguna Street. It's a discreet stucco-ized
Victorian absolutely re-created through alternate
actualization of the original Victorian Image.

Sophistication, but easy sophistication. Where can I
find it for my living space?

We live a very quiet respectful life style on States
Street. We expect our best tenants to appreciate
that mental setting, and then to make the
complete decision to rent in our Canyon View 3-unit
complex.

Challenge: Buy out the "dog lady" and "Don" who
live below. Move down there and create a walkout
garden complex. Eventually sell off the upper
units as part of an exclusive 5-condo complex
"Canyon View."

My Garden

A Sycamore tree. That's what Miguel told me last Wednesday. That little "fern" I transplanted from the middle retaining wall has come to life and grown 7 inches!

Miguel says that Sycamores get to be very big trees. I wondered where I could eventually locate this tree on our property.

Get more critical over what, when, and how much I read. Knock away more of the negative news, the too-busy news.

Substitute "Peace and Quiet," as in the form of leisurely creation in my chosen field, in political advisory or as a public San Francisco advocate. Do it through my writing, photographs, and other creative/practical arts.

I wonder if the Catholic Church still requires "Confession."

"Hole in the Wall"
A South of Market Dive

At least three

And where was I?

Sensuous Michael and David.

Hand and body dances from us all.

Multiple massage and masseurs.

Music to unwind a tight up crowd.

Total success!

How wild can we afford to be?

Who will best adapt on this planet?

Hey, let's set everything to "Automatic."

Let's focus on a sanity beam and follow it.

Bon Voyage

Black Beetle Terror

This was our problem tenant's black motorcycle. He also painted our rental flat Black, all Black!
Morning. Seven-ish.

BAROOM, BAROOM   BAROOM.   BDOMM B   D   o
MM BDOMMBDOMMBDOMM........ BAROOMMMM.
BDOMMBDOMMBDOMM........ BAROOMMMM.

Ohh oo, Alarm set for 7:30. It's Awake and rumbling. Hope it's gone soon. I'll live thru it I guess.
Sounds sick to me. Bad digestion?
Holes in the pipes?
Finally he moves on down the street.
Peace. For now.

Nighttime.

Is it 11?
Is it 2 A.M.? .. 4 A.M.? Just woke
We're up again. It's come back! **Barroom, baroombaroom...**
Or is it leaving?
BAROOM   BAROOM.
BDOMM. B   D M M
BDOMMBDOMMBDOMM........ BAROOMMMM.
BDOMMBDOMMBDOMM........ BAROOMMMM.
..it's leaving now...

The BLACK BEETLE and its owner needs some medical attention. Better breathing, lubricating, repairing. Maybe a simple accelerator depression will set its choke right, and then it can warm up while it is going up or down the hill.

Hope it (he) sees a doctor soon so it can feel better. The neighbors and I will be in a much better state of mind. Everyone will be happier, including black beetle....

Bless you and good health....Your neighbors.

----

3 Fine Ladees

"You're the most polite person I've ever run in to here." I said.

She assumed I had the right away because in my hands was a piece of coconut cream pie and a latte.

"No, you come on through," I said.

Later, with me at my table soaking up the interior sunlight, very comfortable, two of the ladees sat down at the next table. Ladee two comments that I'm taking up a l o t o f space i n my corner angled positioning. We laugh and agree that there is plenty of space for all.

A quick interested glance from her to my cream pie...I guard it with my hands. It's greatly admired by all.

We talk. They leave for the Central outdoor table and in a moment I'm invited to join them outside. I jump up and do.

Ladee one: San Jose Lisa. Leather coat. Prop design and execution for a San Jose civic light theater.

East Bay Ladee t w o : Edits for suburban East Bay papers. Loves it! (Takes lots of attention and insight to do that.)

We share "Korea," "The C a s t r o" and our professional energies.

"G" joins us and the collective conversation shifts into their very active lesbian connection to Bay Area professional and social life. I'm starting to get a new source of lesbian insights!

So....

Ladee two knows Hilda at Magic Theater, who undoubtedly knows John...

I write a hello note on my card for personal delivery).*"Hilda, please say a BIG hello to John from Rob Tackes."* Wonder w h a t t h a t w i l l mean, if anything, in the local theater grapevine!

There's talk of a cozy, personal hot tub-club in a Victorian in the midmission. There's talk of our doing an interactive evening at Josie's Cabaret. Stage center.

The ladees are n e a t, and I get the sense of their vibrant cross current meeting places from San Jose to Pleasanton.

Goodbyes are initiated by me and I remind Ladee two that she reminds me of a major character in last night's screening of KQED's "The Castro"--at the Castro Theater.

I bolt out into the brisk, chilly very late afternoon, fulfilled.

What to Do with My Life?

Is my life art?

Or, am I suffering from delusions that my life with Denis is not on the right track!

Somehow I've got to entrust and evolve to his level, relax, and then do my own thing with the same intensity that he's doing his own things!

Two Jobs I would like:

One: To be $75k a year Ombudsman reporting to Mayor Brown.

Two: To collaborate with an editor and artistic genius. To publish my memoirs, mount my photos and artwork collection regularly in The Chronicle. All my prose and my pictures of San Francisco.

Oh yes, work with the music. Get back into it. Gentility. San Francisco. Seek it out and like it there.

Where's there?

Rent a condo at Park Hill. See if living with 20-40-100 people on all sides, under one roof, is what I really want.

Pacific Heights? I wonder how Denis would get to work.

Isn't there a quality, affordable rental property out there for us? I *think there is, at $4,000 per month.*

Remember...maximize the rents at States Street, buy complete maintenance and management, and be ready to sell or rent and move out.

The Garden Gates Are Open, & I'm "High"

Wow! The gates are open!

My corner garden is open to me.

There's a Big Lady on the bench with me, and I get
into the garden mood immediately.

At the rear are her lady friend and the gardeness
herself.

I meander through and to the back and tell them
about my garden.

I express great thanks for their healthy plants and
for their fabulous San Francisco presentation of
urban floral Art!

Segue

We invite in two young Negroes who have just
lunched at Postrio, a very' downtown French
restaurant. One thinks I'm a dancer *(just because I am
slightly but nicely" high")*. They too, feel good here.

A bit later, Big Lady and I agree on the wisdom of
privatizing and taxing all drugs worldwide to "stop the
madness of waste."

Big Lady responds knowingly to my question:
"Why are these plants so happy?" "Fertilization" she
says, "Fertilization."

Masturbation and Marijuana
The New Sacraments

Why the Social and Religious organizations of previous millennia will be replaced by necessary creations of the 3rd millennium (CE).

I stepped out of a dream, and the dream was madness. The old ways were destroying my mind, life and all the life around me.

Progress was breathing its last hurrah and (other) evil things were threatening to take over the world.

How we can reach a better safer awareness for the 21st century!

Replace old think with the 2 sacraments given to us by god (us), to save humanity's existence on Earth, and to create peace and happiness as the basis for a new World.

Let's straighten our planet first.

All Masturbate,

All Ingest Marijuana,

Live life anew.

Beach Day

Sitting here, now at home e a t i n g a carrot
and some walnuts. Very substantial, I presume
h e a l t h y for me as a snack.

What a late afternoon I have had at Land's End!

A power circle, an old friend, the sea.

Mozart is playing now, and the late afternoon's
filtered sun continues to flow through the
greenery outside my windows.

Temperature 68 degrees and calming.

Yes, a five star day at the beach. Radiant lights -
the color power spot.

Four dimensions - the incoming surf.

Just another special day in S a n Francisco.

PART FOUR

SOME OF MY MOST FAVORITE THINGS

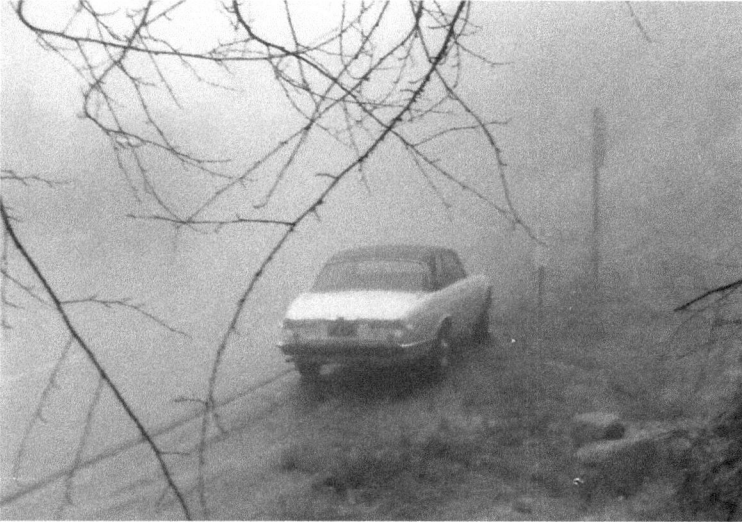

A foggy dream in my '76 Jaguar.

45. CARS I HAVE LOVED

Here are some fond memories of the automobiles in my life. You can see photos of most of these cars on my website (desertmusebooks.com).

My family had a two door 1939 Plymouth that my dad bought for $900 in 1939 just before the war started when I was 2 years old. We drove that car until 1951. All our trips to Wisconsin were made in that car. We always drove Route 14, the Northwest highway. Half way to Delavan there was a huge round metal gas storage tank by the side of the highway that we dubbed "The Crystal Ball." It appeared to us kids that the ball changed sides of the highway as we rounded the bend. It was quite the treat to see the ball on every trip.

Friday nights we stopped at the half way point at restaurant in Crystal Lake. Their Friday Fish Fry was a major treat. When I was twelve I noticed the condom dispenser in their bath room. For a quarter you could get a pack of several condoms. I initially wanted to experiment with one but I was afraid that the family would hear the workings of the dispensing machine. Eventually I did succeed in purchasing a pack.

Dad taught me to drive in Delavan. My first test was to back out of our Delavan driveway and then drive down our gravel road to where it dead ended in a swamp. I completed a turnaround into a neighbor's driveway and successfully returned the car to our cottage. My first big successful trip was to drive my mother the three miles to town on county trunk O.

In 1951 Dad bought a 1950 Oldsmobile. We now had a four door car for the first time. It was a gift from my father to make it easier for mom to enjoy a little more comfort in her last days.

In 1957 at the end of my junior year in college I purchased my first car, an Italian designed 1953 Studebaker coupe. Stick shift, beautiful and low slung. I paid $600 for it, $300 of which was borrowed. Before long I realized that I had bought a "lemon," but I kept car until 1963. The oil consumption was so horrendous that I needed to stock quarts of oil in the trunk so I could top off the oil every time I bought gas.

My second used car was a 1958 Plymouth sports sedan. It had a two tone tan and green color and push button power steering that was so sensitive that I could steer the car with my little finger. Eventually the repair bills made me vow to never buy a used car again.

Continuing my quest to have something a little bit different yet practical, I purchased a new 1965 Toyota Corona. This was the first year that the Japanese started exporting cars to challenge the VW Beetle and the French Renault. They were about $1,500 new at the time, but I only had to pay $1,200 for my new cream colored, four door Corona because it was based on last year's model. It had a classic look, very well proportioned and a profile similar to the luxury Lincoln Continental of the day, or so I imagined.

My Corona served me well and got me across country all the way to San Francisco in the early seventies. My one disappointment was that the car would often not start in the bitter cold Chicago weather. For several years, we rigged an electrical cord out the second story window of our townhouse and attached it to a dip stick that supposedly kept the engine warm enough to start. The dip stick worked most of the time.

In 1971 I needed a car in San Francisco that was new, dependable and different. I decided on a Nissan 240Z, a sleek, affordable sports car. No sooner had I made a deposit and ordered the car, I came down with debilitating hepatitis. My income and job were in jeopardy and I successfully appealed to the Nissan dealership and they thankfully cancelled my sale.

I then lowered my sights, and was considering a Jeep as a different statement, but decided on an 8 cylinder American Motors Gremlin. It was a two-door sedan, golden bronze with lots of power. It was a curious car and unusual with its abrupt and stumpy rear end.

My most exciting event with the Gremlin happened one afternoon as I was pulling into my garage on Alpine Terrace. I eased on the gas pedal and began to slowly pull in and suddenly the accelerator locked and the car lunged 15 feet at top speed into the concrete retaining wall of the garage. I frantically tried to turn off the ignition but it was too late. The hood jumped up, I ground to a halt and smoke started coming up from the engine. I was all shook up but not injured. The body shop was able to repair the front end, believe it or not.

In 1975 my real estate staff thought that I should have a car befitting my new status as president of my brokerage. I fell in love with a 1976 Jaguar SJC coupe on display in the showroom. The look was stunning with a cream color and a black leather hard top. The profile displayed a tasteful very narrow maroon stripe. I bought it. My staff and I were pleased.

Here is something lighthearted about my vanity license plate "I RT I." My idea was to bracket my initials, but others saw it as a double ego statement. Herb Caen, premier San Francisco gossip columnist, writes in his column about what he thought it meant:

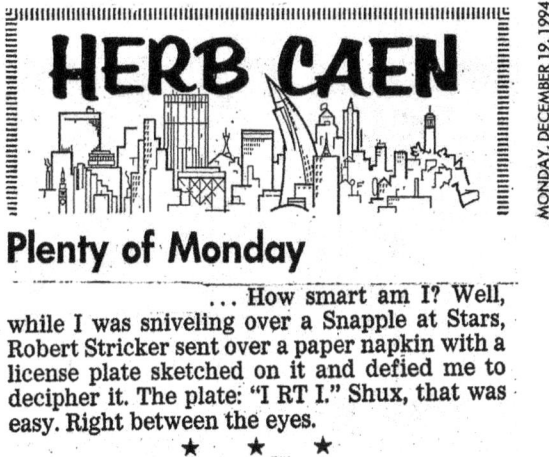

HERB CAEN

MONDAY, DECEMBER 19, 1994

Plenty of Monday

... How smart am I? Well, while I was sniveling over a Snapple at Stars, Robert Stricker sent over a paper napkin with a license plate sketched on it and defied me to decipher it. The plate: "I RT I." Shux, that was easy. Right between the eyes.

★ ★ ★

In 1980 after I closed my brokerage offices I decided to get more practical and I purchased a four-door silver Nissan Sentra. I loved that car. I drove it for many years until one afternoon after smoking a bit too much grass, and having a bit too much hysterical conversation at the Café Flore, I headed to my car and couldn't find it. A week went by searching the streets and I called the police to help. No one found my car, so I leased another car and collected insurance on the Sentra. Shortly after signing the lease contract, I was driving up lower 17th street, just north of Castro Street, and saw my car! It was too late. I did get to visit the auto holding area to take a few possessions out of the trunk. What a disappointment to lose my loved Sentra. For two years thereafter I decided to lease a Nissan Altima. The car was fine but when I turned it in the leasing company they hit me hard to pay for minor scratches.

In the year 2000 I researched on line the new Japanese <u>2001 Prius Hybrid</u>. The car had not yet been approved for sale in the United States but in the autumn of 2000 my reserve order from a San Francisco dealer became a reality. I now was the excited owner of one of the first hybrids in the City and the country. I drive this gas saver in Palm Springs to this day. It has been a joy to drive. I now refer to it as a *soon-to-be classic!*

46. NOSTALGIA – EXPLORING CHICAGO IN THE 1940s & 1950s

We neighborhood kids hung out together on the streets a lot, doing nothing much but innocent talking and playing street games. In summer, we played softball in the cinder lots nearby. In winter, we played and slid on the Ice in the streets. Not to my liking was hanging around on those cold days with relatives in the alley when an auto needed fixing. My perceived poor reaction when playing any sports made me reluctant to be around outside when a game came together. I preferred my radio serials, homework and other more solitary pastimes.

Occasionally I would have the extra money to splurge on a banana split. The sign outside said "Georges Café" and early on I asked what that word café meant, which was French, no less. It meant coffee shop or restaurant. George and his son were smart enough to move to California in 1948 as part of the neighborhood exodus after the war. Café's, I would discover, were to be important getaways for me in the future.

In addition to my visits to the Museums and the Beaches, I found myself exploring the city on my bike. I remember one long ride I took heading North on Western Avenue. At one point, I noticed that the street started sloping up. This was the first time I had experienced anything other than the totally flat ground that I thought the entire city was built on. (It was built on a dried-up lake bed.)

A school tour to the Bowman Dairy Company fascinated me, because at close range, I saw the milk and the bottles as they moved meticulously along the moving, bottling lines.

I had that same feeling when I went on trips with my uncle Art to Chicago's North Shore. Evanston and Wilmette were a whole new world of beauty and mystery and affluence. I would find myself up there more and more as I grew up.

My boyfriends and I would often go bike riding to the far Northwest Side of Chicago. We biked to the forest preserves and rode our bikes up and down on the huge mounds of earth that were being prepared for the first "super highways. We would go to the top of the mounds, and then with utter abandon, speed on down.

In my early teens, we went to theatrical and sporting events around town. Drag races were big in those days. One time we were at Soldier Field, in seats close to the auto action, but the noise and the cinders and the experience were a turn-off to me.

I remember another late-night performance at the big auditorium amphitheater where we saw *Hellzapoppin'* with Olson and Johnson. It was a huge old fashioned vaudeville type extravaganza. We were in the highest farthest cheapest seats in the building. The dirty jokes and a show went on and on, until Midnight. I wanted to get out of there and go home and go to sleep.

Riverview amusement park was a real cultural asset to the city of Chicago. It opened in 1904 and entertained over 200,000,000 people through its lifetime. It boasted over 120 rides, including 6 roller coasters, and was a fun spot for all Chicagoans. In 1967 the park closed and was replaced by a light industrial commercial center. What a shame!

Speaking of parks that we enjoyed as kids, I went to Brands Park often. This was our neighborhood park only three blocks away. On Christmas Eve 1946, my brother Tommy and I went over there to ice skate on the ball field that they flooded each winter. While skating, I fell and hit my head on the ice and became extremely woozy and disoriented, so I had to rely on Tommy to lead me home. I was still able to rationalize and felt confident, because Tommy had just turned seven he was now at the "age of reason," I figured he would understand how to get me home safely, and he did. That Christmas Eve I wound up opening my presents, still bundled up and in poor condition from the fall.

At school I was scoring A's in all my subjects and was secure knowing that I could not be criticized for doing less than perfect. Many Sundays after Mass at St. Francis Xavier, my name would appear on the bulletin acknowledging my top grades. Being bashful, I was somewhat embarrassed with the attention it brought from the people milling around after church services, but secretly I was proud.

47. HOLLYWOOD AND THE MOVIES

One early evening in 1945 I was accompanying my grandma to a movie at the Fox Theater. My parents reminded me to take special care of her because she was "a widow now 65 years old and more vulnerable to falling." I held on to her arm as we walked along the torn-up sidewalks on Belmont Avenue on our way to the theater. The street was being widened and the streetcar tracks were being taken out. The city was installing overhead dual wires, narrowing the sidewalks and preparing for the switchover to the new electric buses. We had to dodge the sidewalk framing where the new concrete still needed to be poured.

We arrived at the theater to see what turned out to be an adult movie and one that I did not understand. It was *The Hairy Ape* by Eugene O'Neil, and the story was beyond me. There was a distinctly hellish scene with William Bendix stoking the fiery furnaces, sweating, shoveling. He appeared to be in Hell. It was scary as Hell.

Another time in the mid-1940s, while watching a typical Hollywood fantasy musical at the Fox Theater, I was shocked to see my uncle Art running up the aisle shouting out loud, ranting about how crazy and unreal the situations were on the screen. Only years later did I understand what was going on, and that he was annoyed with the unreal escapism (and propaganda?) that Hollywood was presenting to the public.

In addition to many Westerns I began to see more adult films that often mystified me at my young age. One of these films was *For Whom the*

Bell Tolls with Gary Cooper and Ingrid Bergman. It took place in Spain during their civil war. People in the big houses had food to eat while thousands of Spanish republicans were dying of hunger outside the gates. I just could not understand why the rich people did not share their food with the starving people. I had only been privy to my small world where all the neighbors had the same standard of living, and enough food to eat. Only much later did I become aware that there was a lot of inequality in the world, and that the privation of war caused horrendous hardship.

I saw a few of the World War II movies that tackled the evil of the Nazis. One film haunts me to this day, and I never have been able to identify it. It had a scary scene in a dark forest where the principal characters were trying to escape the evil Nazis who wanted to kill them. The musical score was a haunting classic which accompanied the action, "Humoresque" perhaps? I had nightmares over and over as a child reliving this scary scenario.

Leave Her to Heaven was shown at the Fox Theater in 1946 and was in glorious color. An image etched in my mind was the image of Gene Tierney outreaching against the sky, hands held high with her dress flowing in the wind. I think she went insane in the movie. Way over my head. I found out later that in real life she did become a mental basket case.

I saw *Golden Earrings* in 1946, and I was told by my family that Marlene Dietrich was a big star, and that I should see it. Up on the screen there she was, in a smoldering scene with Ray Milland. Both were reclining outside by a campfire. Seduction and love (and sex?) was in the air along with a very smoky atmosphere. The rest of the movie was forgettable to me.

In seventh grade my class went to the Esquire Theater to see *Hamlet* with Laurence Olivier. I did not fully understand the story line at that time. However, I will never forget the scene where the dead Ophelia went floating down a river filled with lily pads. I did not imagine why she would kill herself for love. The Esquire Theater was a pure Art-Deco delight, in an area that was clearly more affluent than my neighborhood. It had a certain exciting sophisticated feel to it. I would revisit the area often as I got older, because I sensed that there was something mysterious, sensuous and alluring that I needed to explore.

Another earlier musical, *Meet Me in St. Louis*, also seduced me. The snowy garden scene when Margaret O'Brien smashes the beautiful snow man broke my heart. Judy Garland was beautiful, but I was not necessarily stunned by her presence as I have been of Doris Day's.

With *Romance on High Seas* in 1948, I had my first intense infatuation with a musical. This was a breezy movie in intense Technicolor. It had quick pacing, bright music and energetic acting, and starred Jack Carter, Janice Page, Cuddles Z, and Doris Day, who I immediately fell in love with. After that, Doris Day was my special musical favorite. I looked forward to seeing Doris in any musical. For the next ten years, I saw every one of her films, all the way to *Calamity Jane* and *Love Me or Leave Me*. I thought her role in *Love Me or Leave Me* was the height of her career. My whole world had been opened up to musicals, because they made me feel real good.

In Delavan in the early 1950s I went to the movies at the downtown Delavan Theater, often with my aunt Clara. The musical standouts were *The Band Wagon* and *Singing in the Rain*. I was wowed by the clever musical dance numbers. About that time, I went with my aunt to see the William Inge film *Come Back Little Sheba*. There was a porch swing scene, where Richard Jackal and Terry Moore were doing some very heavy necking. They were breathing heavily, and I became caught up in the sensuality that the hunky blond, Richard Jackal, was passing on to me. I felt a bit uncomfortable sitting with my aunt during this scene. It was arousing me because of that hot man.

Later in my Junior and Senior years in College I became aware of the art film scene and I began to pay special attention to a film's full meanings and their messages. The most thrilling film of that era was *Diabolique*, a French masterpiece that had a shocking scene at the end. A real eye-opener. I ventured alone down to the Auditorium building on south Michigan Avenue to see it. This was my first visit to this iconic building. It has performance spaces for music teachers, and significantly was the site of world renowned Auditorium Theater, that had one of the best acoustics in the country.

Later in life I take great care in choosing films, when to go and what to see. Movies and television assume a secondary role and they took back seat to my career in real estate, and to my active social life. Now, I love catching up with the old black and white films of the 1930s, 1940s and 1950s.

48. MEMORABLE MEN IN CHICAGO

I was fortunate to meet and learn from guys who had entirely different backgrounds. Here are a few more that stand out from my early period in Evanston:

Bernd, I met at "The Bushes," a cruising area just south of the Northwestern campus. He drove a cute black Renault and was terribly disturbed that his father had had him circumcised. I could not fathom his thinking.

Revelle, a black professor, very low key and a gentleman. Surprise! A very big disappointment in the size department.

Bill, a Frat member emeritus. Hot sex. He took me to his fraternity house and I had to jump off the roof to escape being discovered by an incoming clan of brothers. Later in San Francisco we hired his firm to remodel our home.

Chad lived in Chicago with his lover. How soon I was disillusioned. He was an early crush but when we finally got together I found out that he was a dud.

Terry was a grad student at Northwestern. Sweet and charming, but our rendezvous in my attic apartment on Orrington Ave just did not work out.

I met Gabe at an Evanston party. He was a quiet, well-mannered guy who subsequently moved from Chicago to Tempe, Arizona where he went to grad school. I was on my way to California, and I stopped at his place, where we explored Phoenix, and later I spent the night with him on his very narrow bed.

Mike was a sailor from Great Lakes Training station. I met him at one of Jack's coach house parties. Months later, while sitting in my Evanston real estate broker's office, the navy's intelligence staff sauntered in We moved to the conference room where they asked me to sign a statement that Mike was gay. They undoubtedly wanted to expel him from the service. Their story was that he already admitted it and they were gathering information to seal their case. I signed.

We befriended Bill and Rocky, lovers who Denis and I met in the bushes. We attended a party at their house and they recorded some wild action on their 8-millimeter camera. They subsequently moved to San Francisco in the mid-1970s and opened "The Trolley" an ill-fated gay bar at the end of Church Street at 30th St. It turned out that the location at the time was too far from the Castro Street action, and unfortunately, they were inexperienced at running a gay bar.

Paul Hammer was Bill and Rocky's teenage friend and neighbor. I hosted him at my townhouse one evening. He was a total delight, and still living at home. He had such an impressive time with me (and I with him), that he stayed up all night, at his home, creating an intricate ink drawing, that featured my new first name- "ROB." The framed drawing hangs on my wall to this day.

49. A NEW CAFÉ LIFE – CAFÉ FLORE

When we came to San Francisco in 1970, the location of the future Café Flore was an empty lot, adjacent to a Finnish bath house owned by a straight old line San Francisco family. My car had stalled near that empty lot and I was able to come to a stop by pulling into the space. In 1973 a flimsy structure was built and a plant store went in. By 1983 the café was the new tenant. The largely glass and skinny metal construction was perfect for a café, which kept the green theme. Plants abounded inside and out, where there was a wraparound patio protected from street noises by a Plexiglas shield.

In the mid-1980s, I walked in and took a seat inside, and this started a life changing turn of events for me.

I immediately noticed a different set of people enjoying these serene surroundings. I loved it.

From John the professor I learned how to Sautee vegetables in olive oil.

From Uri, I noticed how to have a more laid back approach to living. In Uri's case, he later confessed to me that no day existed when he was not high on cannabis, and that he started each day with it. I was surprised to hear that because I used it sparingly and was an easy high. Uri also revealed that he had been a nationally known disc jockey in Tel Aviv before his trips to India and San Francisco. A number of years later he moved back to Israel and disappeared into the mist.

Dinesh was electric and handsome, but over the years he burned himself out on sex. He gradually became somewhat of a recluse, incorporating music and astrological insights into his life.

A young lady, C.C. read Tarot, and later advertised for a husband in the alternative press. After interviewing several candidates, she chose a German man and moved to Marin County.

Those early years we sometimes smoked dope out on the patio of the Café. Those hippie-like times were slowly slipping away after the waning of the high life that was intimately connected to the Haight Ashbury summer of love. Some of the spinoff people from that set, with similar lifestyles were moving into the Castro, and became one facet of the gay community.

On one occasion after I had returned from Kawai I became a big hit with the Flore crowd, by sharing a fat joint of Maui-Wowi that my Hawaii friend sent back with me. Afternoons were a blast with friendly people coming and going from various venues around the City. Eventually smoking outwardly became a no-no as the café acquired slightly more mainstream credentials.

50. JEROME CAJA - ARTIST EXTRAORDINAIRE

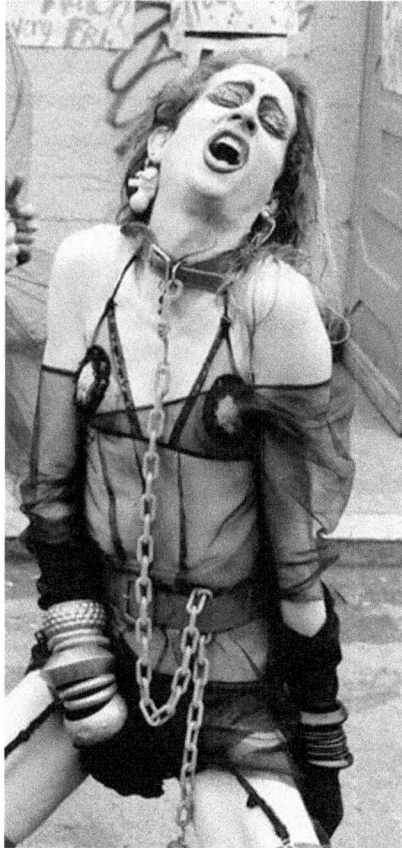

Jerome. The artist in negligee.

Jerome was a San Francisco Art Institute graduate who was an outrageous figure in the alternative club and art scene. He achieved *Enfant Terrible* status in the late 1980s and 1990s, and his passion was creating art in miniature. His art, mostly drug induced, was brilliant and off the wall. These are perspectives that I have always admired. Many of Jerome's works projected a calculated blasphemy, sparked by his spurned, volatile, Catholic childhood in Cleveland.

My first meeting was at his one man show at the Strand Theater, an historic but run down place on Market Street. He was hosting an exhibit of his miniatures in the second story great hall. The eclectic crowd and I were milling around this grand space where the walls were plastered with an unusually large number of Jerome's works. Jerome suddenly appeared, magically, wearing a see-through flowing negligee. I had smoked cannabis and was ready for his outrageousness, I thought. As I approached and embraced him he lit up, flashed a big smile and pinched my nipples the hardest that they have ever been pinched. I was hooked on his specialness.

In the coming months, I purchased several of his less outrageous miniatures, and am proud to display them from time to time. In retrospect, my choices were probably too conservative. A better alternative, from an investment standpoint, would have been to choose his religious art, which dripped with blasphemy, and was an important part of his output. All of his art, astonishingly, contained a hidden layer of imaging and meaning. He was brilliant. He died young.

I did have a relaxed one-on-one encounter and conversation with Jerome, one afternoon at the Café Flore. He sauntered in and I invited him to join me. For the moment he dropped his outrageous public persona and we talked about our shared Catholic upbringing. There the similarities ended. I had walked away easily from my religious roots. Jerome regurgitated his religious experiences with a vengeance through his art. He was a most prolific painter of miniatures. And his works today are in high demand among the cognoscenti.

51. BEACHES!

It was always nice to commune with Mother Nature and to have an opportunity to interact with other gay men in the great outdoors. These diversions helped my cope with my low periods due to HIV.

In the 1970s when Denis and I lived on Alpine Terrace, just down from Buena Vista Park, I would go there and take an uphill walk to the top of the park. In the early years, I could still drive up to the summit, and cruise the hillsides in the many alcoves and undergrowth. Some guys actually got nude there and worked on their tans! An air of mystery and forbidden outdoor sex was the order of the day.

The word was out that there were several nude beaches down the peninsula. Devils Slide was a half hour south of San Francisco, and there was also San Gregorio beach that had caves, and was a bit farther down the coast. It was exciting to go to these beaches, take off your clothes, sunbathe and walk along the sand and cruise and meet new men. These beaches were popular with guys living in the suburbs as well, so the urban and the suburban gay men were able to meet. All were seeking a day of abandon, and excitement in the raw.

Another day trip was to Lake Temescal in the East Bay in Oakland. It was an easy drive over the Bay Bridge, and then, suddenly, you were in a Lake Tahoe setting that was ringed by ridges of thick-forested trees surrounding the area. There was a nice sandy beach for sunning and the crowd was very gay in the early to mid-1970s, but there was more looking than trysting. This spot was the site of the horrific East Bay hills fire, that later burned huge swathes through the forest and destroyed hundreds of homes, although the beach was untouched.

North of San Francisco, there were the Russian river resort communities, with their great laid back outdoor lifestyle. This area had its gay heyday starting in the mid-1970s. The one street downtown was a throwback to the past. Every year during the rainy season parts of all of the downtown area would flood. Another outing was to drive from downtown Guerneville, to the mouth of the Russian River at the ocean. Gay resorts multiplied after the first success of the resort *Fifes,* and city men started to buy up homes as getaways.

Back in San Francisco there was "Roosevelt Beach." It was a grassy area tucked in just below the craggy mountain side on Corona Heights. We rented a home across the street on Roosevelt Way in the early 1980s. For a time, this was a most popular gay space to sun. It was just up the hill from The Castro.

Later in the 1980s and 1990s, the slice of upper Dolores Park became the hottest place for trendy gays to sun, socialize and meet. I went there often to unwind and revel with hot handsome men in their speedos, who had their afternoons free.

There were at least three nude beaches on the north coast of San Francisco and I used them all. Their location just outside the Golden Gate Bridge provided breathtaking views of the Marin County headlands.

Classic "Lands' End" was a hidden rocky cove that sat surrounded by a well-worn path of cruising among the heavy growth on the hillside above. It was well known for many decades by the gay community. The bushes were alive for cruising. Police and park rangers would occasionally make a sweep of the area to keep the action under control.

Baker Beach was located in a cove farther east, and also had a commanding view of the Golden Gate Bridge. There were two alcoves. The more public section had a clothed area and catered to a family crowd at the West End. A "plus" was a nudist optional gay/straight area on the eastern portion. It was a great place to observe beautiful bodies and conduct some discrete socializing. At low tide a sister cove, closer to the bridge was accessible, and was exclusively gay.

I was a "beach bum" of sorts during this era, and I frequently visited all of these beaches, especially in the 90s and through the early 2000s. Most of the nude beaches required a rigorous walk up and down steep slopes. In later years I still traversed them, despite my arthritis, as long as I walked carefully. This was great fun throughout the years, and I never lacked for a generous and full body sun tan.

52. MUSIC!

When I was in college I wanted to expand my musical appreciation, so I started to buy 33 rpm long playing records of serious music, and I made it a point to start going to live concerts. The Ravinia festival in summertime Chicago whetted my appetite for more classics.

In San Francisco I was drawn into the musical world of theater and cabaret that were spinoffs from Denis' artistic interests. Cabaret at the Fickle Fox and concerts at Notre Dame College in suburban San Francisco furthered my education. It was always melodic music, rarely rock or Jazz, although dreamy Jazz does turn me on.

I wake up in the morning and often start singing. Deep bass baritone sounds are easiest for me in the morning. I sing simple melodies from the 1930s, through the 1960s. Mostly just the words from the first lines of music, after which my memory lapses. I easily transform the lyrics into dada sounds, as I fly through my musical ecstasies...

Denis says that my ability to be true to a pitch is amazing, and especially. I am able to adjust my voice instantly into an octave lower if I anticipate trouble hitting a higher note on pitch. He says that my skills at harmonizing and riffing off any music having the least amount of melody are incredible. I fantasize being a backup singer to soloists, divas and choruses.

Another of my specialties is using dada-esque, crazy sounding words and non-words set to melody. I had that same ability at age seven when rattling off a list of rhyming words, one of which turned out to be "fuck." Mom didn't like that one.

I am told that my grandmother was a beautiful singer in the church choir back in Austria and that my grandfather noticed her for that quality, and married her. So, that musical fondness passed on to me. I too was in my church choir and learned some musical tricks early--like pianissimo, and in my high school glee club I was introduced to more musical choral skills.

One of the first connections I had to Denis was that he was an accomplished pianist, and I am proud and revel when attending his concerts and musical events.

Music can bring tears to my eyes, and perhaps my early experiences with lush church music and singing pianissimo for Father Norman at midnight mass at St. Francis Xavier a long time ago got me hooked.

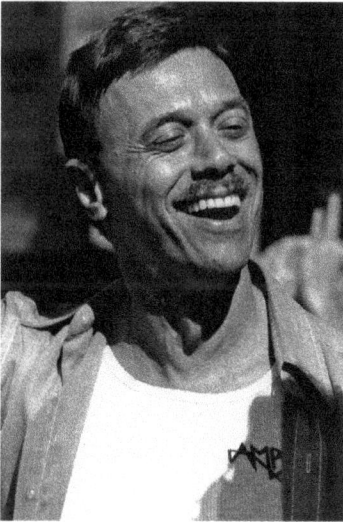

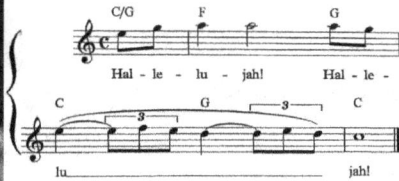

AUTHOR'S NOTES

A fond thank you to Denis Moreen for his ideas and collaboration in getting this memoir into final form for publication.

Many thanks also to my editor, Don Weise, whose guidance was instrumental, and for his advice on the look and focus of my work. Without him, this book would not have been published.

Thanks also to Hjal, who dared me to write this memoir.

The following are a few powerful readings that have piqued my imagination and broadened my insights:

Perfume: The Story of a Murderer. By Patrick Suskind, published 1986 by Alfred A. Knopf.
> *Brings alive the essence of an evil mind.*

1421: The Year China Discovered America. By Gavin Menzies, published 2003 by William Morrow.
> *Hidden history, not readily taught in the USA as typical history.*

The Hare with Amber Eyes: A Hidden Inheritance. By Edmund DeWaal, published 2010 by Picador.
> *A fascinating account of a Jewish family's collection of small Japanese objects, as they were shifted around the globe over turbulent decades.*

Secret Historian: The life and times of SAMUEL STEWARD, professor, tattoo artist, and sexual renegade. By Justin Spring, published 2010 by Farrar, Straus and Giroux.
> *Steward had a life of sexual excess and fetish spanning his long lifetime. He was fortunate to thrive and to survive the oppressive world around him.*

The Discoverers: A History of Man's Search To Know His World and Himself. By Daniel J. Boorstin, published 1983 by Random House.
> *Open the pages anywhere in this account and marvel at details unimagined, about events and ideas that have made our civilization.*

How the Secret Government Works: The Most Explosive Expose. By Dr. Steven Greer, posted 2015 on YouTube. youtube.com/watch?v=oHxGQjirV-c
> *A scary indictment about the future of the earth. Can this be true? Can this trajectory be changed?*

Many thanks to the publishers and photographers who have given permission for me to reprint their works. Most of the photographs in this memoir were taken from the author's personal collection and were originally photographed by him or his family or friends. Images collected from outside sources include the following:

Rush Street: ChuckManCollectionVolume11.blogspot.com, 2015.

Jerome Caja: Rink Foto. LeslieLohman.org, 2009.

Concordia Lutheran Church: Chicago Police Department, 2013.

Belmont Avenue streetcar: LakeviewHistoricalChronicles.org, 2015.

Belmont "L" station: LakeviewHistoricalChronicles.org, 2015.

Belmont Avenue Bridge: Bridgehunter.com, 2016.

"Pair-O-Chutes": ChuckManChicagoNostalgia.wordpress.com, 1999.

"Shoot-the-Chutes": ChuckManChicagoNostalgia.wordpress.com, 1999.

Superman: DC Comics, 1944.

Physique Pictorial: Los Angeles Athletic Model Guild, 1950.

North Avenue Beach House: Tangsphoto.photoshelter.com, 2007.

Lewis Towers: Courtesy of Loyola University Chicago Archives and Special Collections, 1950.

1968 Chicago convention riots: Davesink.com, 2012.